How Psychotherapy Helps Us Understand Sexual Relationships

In this fascinating book, Cherry Potter takes readers on her personal and professional quest for insights into sex, relationships and gender differences. Why do we feel what we feel, and do what we do? What is the impact of 'performance anxiety' on men, and on society generally? Why are women still faking it? Is ubiquitous online porn turning the clock backwards?

The book delves into the work of Freud, Klein, Bowlby and recent developments in attachment theory for insights into our conscious and unconscious fears and desires, and introduces readers to a range of fascinating clients. These include Jeremy, who was so ashamed of his virginity he was unable to have a relationship; Ellie, who repeatedly fell in love with unobtainable men; Kieran, whose fear of abandonment threatened to wreck his gay relationships; Dulcie, who for years had been unable to face the truth that her husband was having multiple affairs; and Lars, who was addicted to online porn and prostitutes. The book shows how the work between therapist and client is a process of learning together, which is at times painful and deeply moving, but can also reflect a renewed vitality and hope for the future, particularly when it comes to talking about sex.

How Psychotherapy Helps Us Understand Sexual Relationships: Insights from the Consulting Room will be of great interest to both the general reader as well as psychotherapists and counsellors.

Cherry Potter is a UKCP-registered psychotherapist, group analyst and couple therapist. She was formerly a writer and film school lecturer, and she has run screenwriting workshops in many countries. She has published three books and many articles about film, culture and relationships. She sees clients at her private practice in Brighton.

"What strikes me is Cherry Potter's openness, how engaging her book is and how much I identify with it. I've no doubt this will be a great book for therapists as well as for people struggling to understand their own sexuality. But I suspect its real value will be for encouraging people to be as honest with themselves as Cherry Potter has been."

Philippa Perry, Psychotherapist, Author, Presenter of *Sex Lies and Lovebites: The Agony Aunt Story* (BBC Four), *The Great British Sex Survey* (Channel 4) and others

"Her writing style is accessible and her knowledge of psycho-analytic theory obvious. I recommend it widely."

Paula Hall, UKCP Accredited Sexual and Relationship Psychotherapist, Founder and Clinical Director of the Laurel Centre, Author, *Sex Addiction: A Guide for Couples and Those Who Help Them*

How Psychotherapy Helps Us Understand Sexual Relationships

Insights from the Consulting Room

Cherry Potter

Routledge
Taylor & Francis Group
LONDON AND NEW YORK

First published 2020
by Routledge
2 Park Square, Milton Park, Abingdon, Oxon OX14 4RN

and by Routledge
52 Vanderbilt Avenue, New York, NY 10017

Routledge is an imprint of the Taylor & Francis Group, an informa business

British Library Cataloguing-in-Publication Data
A catalogue record for this book is available from the British Library

Library of Congress Cataloging-in-Publication Data
A catalog record for this book has been requested

ISBN: 978-0-367-17778-2 (hbk)
ISBN: 978-0-367-17781-2 (pbk)
ISBN: 978-0-429-05764-9 (ebk)

Typeset in Gill Sans
by Apex CoVantage, LLC

For Brian and Danielle and in memory of Stephen

We never have so little protection against suffering as when we are in love; we are never so desolate as when we have lost the object of our love or its love for us.

—Sigmund Freud (1930)

Contents

Preface

It's hard to talk about our own sexual relationships, even in the confidential space of a psychotherapist's consulting room, without omissions, half-truths and lies, even lies to ourselves. How can we be honest in a world where we are all supposed to be sexually and emotionally savvy without the fear of being judged, found inferior or lacking in some way? As a psychotherapist, naturally, I believe that talking is the best way to understand our deepest feelings, however irrational and seemingly full of contradictions. I also know that many of us find talking honestly about our behaviour in our intimate relationships, and particularly our sexual feelings, fraught with embarrassment and even guilt and shame. But for many clients, even if they come for help because they are suffering from anxiety or depression, talking about relationships, including their sexual relationships or lack of sexual relationships, often turns out to be an important part of their therapy. The work of psychotherapy is rarely easy. Yet one of the most heartening things I have learnt is that after we have bitten the bullet and discovered that we can talk about what needs to be talked about, there is a palpable sense of relief and a renewed vitality and optimism for the future.

My aim with this book is to share my attempts to understand some of the complexity of our sexual feelings and the kinds of problems that frequently arise in our sexual relationships. I also love stories. I spent many years as a writer and teacher of film and creative writing before I trained as a psychotherapist. I know how beneficial other people's stories are as a way of helping us to understand our own experiences, feelings and the many dilemmas we face in life. I have included a few stories that illustrate things

I have learned from my own life. But the most important stories in this book are the case studies based on my work with clients in my consulting room. These stories show how my clients and I, together, have tried to understand what's going on in their relationships. How we have tracked back into their past relationships and childhood experiences. How we discovered repeating patterns, compulsive destructive and self-destructive behaviours, and complicated defence systems that may have once served to keep them safe but are now long past their use by date. The stories show how we celebrated moments of insight together, and how we confronted difficult conversations about what it might mean to change. But of course, change has already started; understanding ourselves better is change, letting feelings out is change, for some people discovering that it is possible to trust the intimacy of a relationship, even if that intimacy is a conversation with a psychotherapist, is change.

I have delved into the ideas and research of various psychoanalysts, sexologists, psychologists and sociologists which have helped me to understand some of the complexity of what goes on in our sexual relationships. I have done my best to write about the psychoanalytic ideas in a way that makes them interesting, relevant and accessible.

I don't promise to provide answers to the many questions raised in this book. It is up to each of us to make our own decisions about how we live our lives. My aim is to pass on what I have learnt to readers, to offer ways of thinking and talking about the many dilemmas and choices we all face in our sexual relationships, and hopefully to enable readers to feel less alone with a subject that is all about intimacy and yet, notoriously, leaves many of us feeling isolated and alone.

This book is for professional and training psychotherapists and counsellors who, like me, are interested in sexual relationships. It is also for general readers who are struggling with problems in their sexual relationships. It is about both sexes, for both sexes. I passionately believe women's and men's sexual and relationship liberation depends on both genders, straight or gay, joining the conversation.

Given the confidential and sensitive nature of this topic, I am hugely grateful to my ex-clients who, because they recognised how a book about psychotherapy and sexual relationships might help others with similar problems to theirs, have given me permission to share the stories of the work we did together. They have also advised me about an effective identity disguise, and in some cases contributed valuable insights into the pieces I have written about their therapy. However, there are two exceptions. In Chapter 5 I have written about a woman's group I conducted so long ago that I was unable to track down all the group members. The client I have called Denise is a fictional portrait based on my experience as a group therapist with similar clients. In Chapter 9, the material is particularly sensitive and the clients whose stories I have referred to are fictional representations based on my experience with clients who have suffered from abusive relationships.

1 It all begins in childhood

All sexual relationship stories begin when we begin, in childhood.

Just one sentence in and already I need to pause and take a deep breath. The subject of childhood sexual feelings often arouses deep anxiety, suspicion and even hostility – particularly in an era when we are beset by a seemingly endless flow of headlines about childhood sexual abuse. But talking about childhood sexuality is essential if we are to understand our adult sexual relationships.

One of the biggest controversies surrounding Freud was, and still is, the importance he placed on sex and childhood sexual development in his attempt to understand the human condition. He was aware of the wish to cling on to the fantasy of childhood as a sex-free zone. Nevertheless, his determination to understand the kind of normal neuroses that afflict us all, as well as the more extreme neuroses, inevitably led him into the territory of childhood sexuality.

Alfred Kinsey, the American sexologist, famously hated Freud and anything to do with psychoanalysis. Yet even he reluctantly conceded that sexual development in childhood is 'a prime source of adult patterns of sexual behaviour and of many of the characteristics of the total personality' (Kinsey 1948). He arrived at this conclusion as a result of the huge amount of data he collected in his sexual history questionnaires; by 1948 more than 18,000 men and women had divulged their most intimate sexual secrets. Kinsey and his team of researchers couldn't help noticing connections between the men's and women's accounts of their childhood sexual experiences and their behaviour as adults.

In my work as a psychotherapist, I am often reminded of how feelings we experienced long ago as children worm their way into our intimate adult relationships. The moments in therapy sessions when we become aware of these connections are often deeply moving; something important has risen to the surface. There are many examples of this in my clients' stories which I shall write about later. But first I want to begin with a few stories from my own childhood in the 1950s and 1960s.

My universe back then was a small village in the countryside. This was long before the Internet or mobile phones. Nevertheless, I believe the sheer complexity of what one child, me, went through when I was trying to understand my body, my sexual feelings, my gender and the attitudes of others around me will still resonate. Some aspects of childhood never change.

Some reflections on my childhood anxieties about sex

I remember being aware of sexual feelings in my body when I was very small. My earliest memory is when I was four years old. It is early morning. I am alone in our sitting room that overlooked the village street. My father has left early to catch the bus to the secondary school where he teaches. I am watching my sister, who is three years older than me, greeting her best friend in the street outside and the two of them setting off together on the half-mile walk to the village primary school. I am envious; I desperately want to go to school but I am still too young. I can hear my mother in the kitchen washing up the breakfast things. She thinks I am getting dressed, but my clothes are still in a heap on the chair where she left them. Instead I crouch in front of the electric fire, enjoying feeling the warmth and touching my naked body. I'm alert, listening, in case my mother should come in. It's important that she doesn't see what I am doing.

Thinking about this memory now, I'm puzzled. Why was I so sure that the pleasure I gained from my own body should remain a secret? I don't remember my mother ever reprimanding me for touching myself. At the time I thought this was because she didn't know. At that age I don't remember being worried about what I was doing, just knowing I must be vigilant. My sexual anxiety set in when I was a few years older.

My sister liked playing with dolls and helping our mother, who had suffered from depression on and off since I was born. I felt closer to our father. I was a curious, talkative child and he was always ready to answer my many questions about the world. I was also a tomboy and happiest when I was playing in the nearby woods with the small gang of village children, mostly boys. We built secret camps out of branches and leaves, and one of our favourite games was 'I'll show you mine if you show me yours'. I remember asking my father what the boys' 'thing' was called, and the pride I felt when he told me it was called a penis. I was impressed: the penis was visible, and it also had a name. I also wanted to know why boys had a penis and girls didn't. But I don't remember asking him that. Instead I was left with the troubling thought that being a girl meant I had an absence; being a girl meant I lacked a penis. Yet I felt deep sensations of pleasure that led to a moment of intense satisfaction when I touched myself in a specific place where a penis should be. I was puzzled. But why didn't I ask my parents for an explanation? Why was it that I seemed to know that I should keep this mystery about my body secret?

A momentous event happened when I was seven. My brother was born. He not only displaced me as the youngest member of our family, but he was also a real boy. Had I really been meant to be a boy, but because of secretly touching myself I had inadvertently rubbed my penis away? I didn't know the word for masturbation.

As I write about this, I can almost hear Freud whispering 'penis-envy' in my ear. In a way, he would have been right. I do remember envying boys their penises. But my penis-envy was at least partly due to my ignorance. I was a little girl struggling to make sense of my body, my gender and my sexual sensations at a time when the mysterious private parts between a girl's legs were taboo. Because girls at that time were not told the words for clitoris, labia and vagina; we did not know they existed. But we knew the word for penis, or 'willy' as it was more often called. In the absence of any language to describe the sexual parts of my body or my sexual sensations, I lacked any information to help me understand my own body and reassure me that I was normal. Whilst, somehow, I had learnt that it was normal for boys to play with their penis even if it was bad, I had become anxious and afraid that I was the only little girl in the world who touched herself in this way.

There was only one way, I thought, to find out. One day as we were walking home from school, I asked my best friend. Rosemary ran off laughing, leaving me alone and acutely embarrassed and ashamed. This was something little girls were not supposed to do. I was abnormal. Not long after this, I went to Rosemary's house to ask if she could come out to play. Her mother opened the door and told me sternly that she wanted a word with me. She took me into her scrupulously tidy sitting room and made me stand to attention in front of her. I was frightened; she was enormous, and I was transfixed by the rolls of flesh bulging around her neck. I fidgeted uncomfortably as she informed me that I was a rude, disgusting, dirty little girl and her daughter was not allowed to play with me anymore. I remember running out of the room in tears, my face burning with shame. I couldn't believe Rosemary had told her my secret. Village children knew what not to tell grown-ups.

But still, I didn't ask my father or any grown-up for reassurance. Instead I tried to resolve my anxiety by issuing myself dire threats about all the terrible things that would befall me if I ever touched myself there again. One of the threats was that I would go blind. But why should I think that I would go blind? I have no memory of anyone telling me this. Maybe I picked up the idea from the village boys. It was common at that time for boys to be told they would go blind if they played with their willy. There was no need to threaten girls because we didn't have a penis, therefore we didn't masturbate.

It was many years before I learnt that the pleasure I experienced was because I was touching my clitoris. In the absence of knowing that I even had a clitoris, I remained convinced that I was the only little girl in the world who did what I did; there was something wrong with me. However, despite my increasingly dire threats of self-punishment, including threatening to kill myself if I didn't stop, I failed miserably.

Another time, I was playing in the woods with a boy who was a few years older than me. After we had finished building a camp or damming up a stream or whatever we were playing, he suggested that we should both take off all our clothes, I was to lie down flat on my back and he would lay down on top of me. We lay there for maybe a few seconds, neither of us moved, he stood up and we put our clothes back on. He solemnly informed me that we were to do this every day if we were to get married. We never did it again.

I don't recall feeling anything particularly sexual when this boy lay on top of me. The boy didn't have an erection – not that I knew what an erection was when I was seven. I would guess that he may have seen some grown-ups having sex and our re-enactment through sex play was his attempt to understand what they were doing. I don't believe his actions were sexual molestation. But it is interesting that I still remember the incident after all these years. I suspect it stuck in my memory because I believed what we were doing was rude.

Looking back, I can see how my parents may have prided themselves on being freethinking, liberal-minded people who believed children should be free to roam the countryside without supervision. But they were also subject to the inhibitions they had learnt in their own childhoods. I never saw them naked. They slept together in a double bed, but I was completely unaware they did anything other than kiss and cuddle. If the subject of sex ever came up, and I don't recall that it ever did, I imagine it would have caused awkwardness and avoidance. I recall feeling curious and acutely uncomfortable when I saw my little brother playing with his penis, but my parents ignored it. If they knew their younger daughter masturbated, they never mentioned it.

Their silence left a vacuum which I filled with whatever I could glean from other children. The association between sex, sin, rude, dirty and bad was firmly planted in the minds of all the children I knew. We all knew that anything to do with sex was rude and forbidden, which meant that the games we played in secret in the woods were even more daring and exciting. The effect of this was that, even at a very young age, I was beginning to develop a keen sense of the curiosity and excitement associated with the secret and the forbidden.

My village is just one small example of what I think has the most significant impact on us throughout our sexual lives – our culture and our community's attitudes towards sex.

What Freud and Kinsey told us about childhood sexuality

As early as 1905, Freud published his views on childhood sexuality. He knew sexual life did not begin at puberty (as most people pretended to believe, probably choosing to ignore the fact that, like me, they could remember all sorts of sexual sensations and adventures long before puberty) but soon after birth. Kinsey also realised from his research that 'erections may occur immediately after birth and, as many observant mothers (and a few scientists know), it is practically a daily matter for all small boys, from the earliest infancy and up in age' (Kinsey 1948).

Both Freud and Kinsey talked about how masturbation and sex play is normal for both boys and girls from two years old or younger, and that there is very little difference between a little boy playing with his penis and a little girl playing with her clitoris apart from size. Small children also enjoy showing off their genitals and exploring other children's genitals – hence the game we played as children: 'You show me yours and I'll show you mine'.

Kinsey interviewed a range of pre-adolescent boys who disclosed an extraordinary array of sexual stimuli that had given them erections, such as sitting on warm sand, sitting in church, fast bicycle rides and fast elevator rides, being scared, fear of punishment, being yelled at, urinating, seeing females or sex pictures, viewing yourself nude in the mirror. One of my clients vividly recalled the sexual thrill when he glimpsed the tops of his mother's stockings when he was about six years old. Another told me how he had come across his mother's silk panties on the floor of his parents' bedroom when he was six. He had felt a thrill of excitement. He secretly undressed, pulled on her panties and climbed onto a chair to view himself in her dressing table mirror.

Freud would not have been surprised by these accounts of what excited young boys. He had noticed how the rhythmic movement of trains was sexually stimulating to boys, and he even speculated about whether this was why so many boys said they wanted to be train drivers when they grew up. He also noticed how some strong emotions, including unpleasant ones such as intense apprehension, fear of punishment, or actual punishment can cause young boys to want to touch their genitals and to experience a sensation that Freud rather quaintly described as like 'a nocturnal emission with all its bewildering consequences' (1905). He became interested in how the sexually exciting effect of emotions that are in themselves unpleasant, such as fear, horror, or punishment, persists in some people throughout their adult lives, and he went on to make a connection with sadomasochism. And of course, his interest in childhood sexual fantasies that feature our opposite sex parent became central to his formulation of the famous Oedipus complex (more about Oedipus later).

The psychoanalyst Melanie Klein devoted much of her life to working with infants and young children. She agreed with Freud that children's early sexual experiences were normal and very important to their development. She also noted that young children's sexual relations with each other include 'looking, touching, performing excretion in common' (Klein 1928).

Children's sex play is normal; it is part of their other play and it wouldn't be problem for children if it wasn't for the disturbing, sometimes frightening and often bewilderingly contradictory messages they pick up about sex from the world of older children and grown-ups. In recent years, children also must contend with information and misinformation about sex they find in Internet searches and the deluge of disturbing sexual images on social media and Internet pornography.

The response of some adults when they see a child masturbating, showing off their genitals or engaging in any kind of sexual activity can be extreme. They become agitated, disturbed and even enraged; they demand that the child stops fiddling with themselves and slap the child to make it stop. One famous story from Freud is the case of Little Hans, aged three, whose mother threatened him that if he didn't stop playing with his 'widdler' (his name for his penis), she would send him to the doctor to have it cut off (Freud 1909).

Some adults, mothers, fathers, older siblings or whoever is caring for the child, have an opposite reaction; they lose all sense of boundaries and become narcissistically involved in the child's sexual activities, persuading themselves that they are only playing with the child when in fact they are stimulating themselves by engaging with the child's sex play. And some grown-ups or older children ignore the child's boundaries and autonomy completely. Many people never recover from the trauma of the sexual things done to them as children. In short, all children learn very early in their lives that society is awash with bewildering mixed messages, ranging from fascination to disgust, when it comes to anything to do with sex.

My world as a teenage girl becomes more sexually confusing

I went to the girls' grammar school in the local town when I was 11. I was still trying to work out exactly what sexual intercourse entailed. One day a girl in my form explained to me that the man must lay on top of the naked girl and put his thing inside her. But beware! Her mother had warned her that if a man saw you naked, sunbathing on a secluded beach for instance, the man would turn wild. Like a wild animal, he would have to have sexual intercourse with you because he wouldn't be able to control himself. Men were like this. This is why you must never let a man see you naked unless you are married.

I didn't believe her mother's story about men turning into wild animals. But it was around this time that I was seized by a new anxiety. I became afraid to go to sleep at night in case I died. I was so anxious about dying that I thought I was ill, although the doctor couldn't find anything wrong with me. It didn't occur to me to tell my parents that I was afraid of dying. Instead one night I found a solution on my own. I took a torch, pencils and a sheet of drawing paper to bed, and under the sheets I shakily drew a picture of a naked woman with a naked man lying on top of her. The image of the man was levitating just above her with his erect penis jutting down to touch her pubic area. When I finished the drawing, I felt a surge of relief. Now I had experienced sexual intercourse, the most important thing in a woman's life, I remember thinking, now it would be alright if I died. I climbed out of bed, hid the drawing and went to sleep. The next day I made a miraculous recovery and returned to school.

Looking back, I can see that in my child's mind I was struggling to conquer my anxiety about two of the most important things in life: sex and death. Not only were the two in some way connected in my child's mind, but relieving my anxiety about sex helped me overcome my fear of death.

For the next few years, the main topic of conversation in the school breaks was the boys who went to the nearby boys' school, and what girls had to do to attract boys. Nice girls were meant to be pretty and passive. Girls who were bold, flirtatious or sexually active were called 'slags'. Sex for a nice girl was okay above the waist but not below, and satisfying the boy's sexual needs was of primary importance so long as you resisted his inevitable attempts to 'go all the way'. The subject of satisfying our own sexual needs, apart from kissing, was hardly mentioned. As girls, we were supposed to gain all the satisfaction we needed through our power to attract the most beautiful boy and show him off as our boyfriend.

As I became increasingly obsessed with my appearance and boys, my previously close relationship with my father changed. I was desperate for his reassurance that I was attractive and pretty. But he appeared to lose interest in me and stubbornly ignored my many ploys to get his attention. I now suspect that, like many fathers of teenage girls, he was disturbed by his own feelings in response to his daughter's burgeoning sexuality. Rather than risk responding inappropriately, he shut me out. I would have to look elsewhere for my reassurance.

I left home at 17 and went to art school. It wasn't long before I became embroiled in a secret love affair with a married lecturer twice my age. Heartbroken and guilt-ridden, I fled to London to a new art school and a new era. The London art schools in the late 1960s were hotbeds of free sex and revolutionary politics. The boys planned the revolution; our role as girls was to look pretty in our white lipstick and Mary Quant miniskirts and service the boys and our male tutors' sexual desires. The impact on me was not good. By my 19th birthday I was seriously confused and depressed.

Judging by the fact that my art college employed its own psychotherapist, I wasn't the only messed up student in those turbulent times. His name was Dr Higgins; he was a Freudian and I saw him once a week. We talked about my relationship with my father and a fear that had taken hold of me that it was me my father secretly sexually desired, not my mother, which caused me terrible feelings of guilt and shame that I should even imagine such a terrible thing. I had informed Dr Higgins in my first visit that I knew all about Freud and I didn't want him slotting me into some Freudian pigeonhole. In fact, I knew very little about Freud, certainly not enough to know that these confused feelings about my parents fitted rather neatly into Freud's theory of the Oedipus complex.

It took me nine months before I mustered the courage to confess another cause of my sexual anxiety. I told him that I had masturbated from an early age. This was the first time, since my ill-fated attempt to tell my friend Rosemary when I was seven, that I had told anyone that I masturbated. I dared to glance at the middle-aged man who was sitting opposite me in his pinstriped suit with his legs crossed, listening carefully. I thought I detected a frown, but I ploughed on. I told him that although I enjoyed it when a man came inside me during sex, I was very worried about not having a 'proper vaginal orgasm'. He uncrossed his legs, stroked his chin, crossed his legs again, cleared his throat and carefully explained to me that he was most concerned; I had become stuck in a sexually immature, regressive phase because I masturbated. This was why I wasn't experiencing a vaginal orgasm. When I left his consulting room that day I was devastated, convinced that I was fundamentally deficient as a woman. I never went back.

In this brief account of my childhood and teenage years, I have touched on a few of the many fears and insecurities about our sexual feelings that still come up, as we shall see, in my work with adult clients. But first I want to go back to the roots of some of the frankly wrong-headed ideas about female sexuality that had such a devastating impact on me as I was growing up.

Women struggle to reclaim their sexuality

I hate to think how many women like me were told by well-meaning but misguided Freudian psychoanalysts that they were sexually inadequate or immature. It wasn't that Freud didn't know about the clitoris. As we have seen, he was aware that girls as well as boys masturbate. Probably because he was a man of his times, he was fixated on the superiority of the penis and convinced that penetration must be necessary to enable a woman to experience his so-called mature orgasm. To support his belief, he formulated the idea that at puberty young girls make an important transition to womanhood, which entails giving up their attachment to their clitoris in favour of their vagina. Many girls had been punished by their parents or nannies for masturbating when they were children, or were, like me, unaware they even had a clitoris. However, according to Freud, failure to complete the 'transition' successfully results in a 'masculinity complex', lesbianism and a whole variety of so-called hysterical neuroses. Women who had difficulty reaching an orgasm through vaginal penetration alone, despite enjoying vaginal penetration and experiencing no difficulty reaching a clitoral orgasm, were led to believe their orgasms were not 'the real thing' or they were frigid. As late as the 1970s, lesbianism was still a shameful secret and 'frigid' a term of abuse – better to fake it than risk the shame of being revealed as frigid.

Even if Freud's so-called mature femininity – the ability to have a vaginal orgasm – was achieved without neurosis, he believed that a 'sense of inferiority' to men was the inevitable consequence of being a woman. As he put it: 'After a woman has become aware of the wound to her narcissism [her lack of a penis], she develops, like a scar, a sense of inferiority' (Freud 1925). I think it is worth pointing out that he did not say women were inferior; he said that at a deep level they *felt* inferior. I think many women do feel inferior sexually, but not for the reasons Freud talks about.

As early as the 1920s, three prominent women psychoanalysts – Karen Horney, Helen Deutsch and Melanie Klein – were questioning Freud's patriarchal theories about female sexuality. Horney questioned Freud's assertion that women feel their genitals to be inferior to a man's and cited this as an example of male narcissism. She realised that a problem for girls was society's assumptions about the superiority of men, and pointed out that just as Freud's theories about female sexuality were rooted in male fantasies, our whole civilisation is a male-dominated civilisation. But at least Freud had put the subject of sex – the impact of repressed sexuality and the negative attitudes towards sex in society – on the agenda, including the prevalence of negative social attitudes towards female sexuality.

Deutsch shifted the emphasis to the mother-daughter relationship. She thought the problem of women's self-esteem was rooted in their ambivalent relationships with their mothers and the conflict faced by many mothers between meeting their own narcissistic needs and attending to the needs of their daughters.

Of these three women, Melanie Klein has had the most enduring impact on the future of psychoanalytic thinking. She was the first to place primary importance on what she realised was an extremely complex and deeply ambivalent love-hate relationship between mothers and their infants, both boys and girls, in the first few years of life. Klein's work was an early precursor to attachment theory and the wealth of research we now have looking at the impact of the kind of love (or lack of love) babies and toddlers receive from their mothers or care-givers on the kind of relationships they form in later life. However, sadly, most male and female psychoanalysts for much of the 20th century continued unquestioningly to accept Freud's controversial theories of women's sexuality.

To add to the general muddle of what it means to be female, Freud also reputedly came up with this much quoted statement: 'The great question that has never been answered, and which I have not yet been able to answer, despite my thirty years of research into the feminine soul, is: What does a woman want?' I have always thought this to be one of Freud's more silly quotes. Why should the issue of what a woman wants be any more mysterious than what any of us wants, male or female? But we must not underestimate the power of words, particularly words uttered by a powerful patriarch such as Freud, in perpetuating the mystification of women.

Freud is reputed to have said this to Princess Marie Bonaparte, who was one of his patients and later became a psychoanalyst herself. What Bonaparte wanted was a vaginal orgasm. One of her reasons for consulting Freud was her failure to achieve 'the real deal' during sexual intercourse. Presumably Freud told her pretty much what Dr Higgins had told me. Bonaparte's reaction was to decide that 'the problem' was biological: the distance between her clitoris and her vagina must be too great. Consequently, she found a doctor to surgically move her clitoris closer to her vagina. The operation was unsuccessful (Moore 2009).

Bonaparte remains an early example of the legions of women who turn to surgery as a way of resolving feelings of inadequacy as women. One of the more bizarre current trends is surgery to reduce women's labia. How do women know their labia are ugly? They are comparing their vulvas with the women in the ubiquitous Internet pornography that has become a model for many modern young women for how they are expected to look and behave sexually to be desirable to men.

Luckily for me, in the mid-1970s books like *The Myth of the Vaginal Orgasm* and *The Hite Report, A Nationwide Study of Female Sexuality* began hitting the bookshops. Because of feminism, young women everywhere were joining what we called consciousness-raising groups. These were spontaneous, self-help groups where women got together regularly to talk about every aspect of our experience, including taking control of our sex lives – actually taking control was another matter. But at least the idea of getting to know our own bodies and doing what turned us on, not just what we thought turned men on, was being discussed. What we were beginning to realise was that our feelings about ourselves, our bodies and relations between men and women cannot properly be understood without considering the cultural context and society's attitudes towards sex, gender roles and power relations between the sexes.

The aim of these early women's groups was change. We wanted to change our lives, we wanted to feel better about ourselves as women, we wanted an end to the patriarchal social structure, and we wanted equality with men. We assumed that if feminism achieved its aims for gender equality in society, the sexual fulfilment that we desired as women would automatically follow. In other words, if women were no longer treated as inferior by society and by men, we would feel better about ourselves and the so-called wound to women's narcissism and deep sense of inferiority would magically disappear.

Looking back as a psychotherapist at those exciting early days of feminist reawakening, I realise that we had no real grasp of the complexity and the difficulty of changing attitudes in the most intimate sphere of sexuality.

Despite the many advances in gender equality over recent decades, many women today, including women who are successful at work and socially, are still confused and uncertain about their sexual needs and still don't know how to talk to their partners about what they want. Many women still suffer from deep feelings of inferiority, worthlessness and self-hatred. In fact, in the highly sexualised climate of the 21st century, the impact of social media, the beauty industry and the easy availability of pornography, feelings of worthlessness and self-hatred have intensified for men as well as women. But I think the impact on men is different, as we shall see.

2 Big changes, entrenched attitudes

The sexologists discovered the truth: Why did we forget?

'Let's talk about sex', was the caption on the billboard posters for *Kinsey*, a film that came out in 2005 about Alfred Kinsey, the controversial American sexologist. But why this sudden interest in a sexologist who had died half a century earlier, long before most of the film's 21st-century audience was born? Was Kinsey's story just an excuse for another nostalgia biopic with a touch of sex to spice it up? Or did his work still have relevance for modern generations? I was puzzling over these questions for an article I was writing for the *Guardian* newspaper when a colleague handed me Kinsey's biography by Jonathan Gathorne-Hardy (2005). Soon I was deeply ensconced in Kinsey's research.

As early as 1935, Kinsey was challenging society's ignorance about human sexuality. He upset the status quo with his controversial view that delaying sexual experience until marriage was psychologically harmful. He also devised a scale for measuring sexual orientation – 0 for exclusively heterosexual and 6 for exclusively homosexual – and announced that his research findings suggested that many normal human beings were somewhere in between. This was a brave thing to do at a time when homosexuality was still a crime. But Kinsey's most celebrated works were his two groundbreaking reports: *Sexual Behaviour in the Human Male* (1948) and *Sexual Behaviour in the Human Female* (1953). Not only did he challenge prevailing assumptions about human sexuality, but he also threw a spanner in the works of Freud's notions about female sexuality.

Kinsey had carried out gynaecological tests on 900 women, and the results established conclusively that the vagina had practically no nerve endings; 86 percent felt little or nothing when probed. He came to the controversial conclusion that although the vagina took part in general spasms and convulsions at orgasm, the vaginal orgasm was a biological impossibility, a myth. Kinsey even discovered that although the penis is bigger it is not more sensitive than the clitoris, in fact the area that is tactilely sensitive is greater in the female genital area. As for masturbation, Kinsey discovered that most women who masturbated used clitoral stimulation. Fewer than 20 percent included some form of vaginal penetration, and then only because they felt they should.

How interesting: it was Kinsey, a man, who was the first to suggest that the vaginal orgasm was a myth that had evolved as an expression of male dominance. He even suggested that men needed to believe that it was essential for a woman to have a penis inside them to orgasm because it made men feel necessary and important.

My initial response to reading all this was amazement – not because these ideas were new to me, but because I had no idea that Kinsey had discovered so much about women's sexuality as early as the 1950s. What had gone wrong? Why hadn't *Sexual Behaviour in the Human Female* changed the lives of women of my mother's generation and consequently of future generations? Why hadn't my mother told me about my body and the clitoris? And what about Dr Higgins, the Freudian psychotherapist I had seen when I was a sexually confused 19-year-old student? Why had he informed me with such superior, male authority that women who didn't have vaginal orgasms were sexually immature? Hadn't he bothered to read Kinsey's research?

Perhaps this is not so surprising. *Sexual Behaviour in the Human Female* was first published in one of the most morally conservative decades of the 20th century. The 1950s was a time when women, like my mother, who had discovered a real sense of pride, fulfilment and sexual freedom when they had worked alongside men during the war, were now expected to stay at home and gain all the fulfilment they needed through their role as housewives and mothers. In 1947 came the publication of *The Modern Woman: The Lost Sex*, a hugely influential bestseller by Ferdinand Lundberg, a reactionary sociologist, and Marynia Farnham, an old-school psychiatrist. Together they had used the full weight of their professional scientific status to make the devastating claim that society was suffering from an epidemic of psychologically disordered women that was having a terrible effect on men as well as on the fabric of society. According to them, this epidemic was caused by women going out to work, and feminists who were claiming masculine power: 'Women should not seek to imitate men but to accept their femininity through subordination to their husbands and the joyful acceptance of motherhood.' Their message was that normal, feminine women should remain virgins until they are married and then live passively through their husbands and children. The result was that single women were stigmatised as unfulfilled spinsters. Housewives like my mother, who felt isolated and trapped at home, were diagnosed with depression and routinely treated with electric shock therapy. Only the wealthy had access to psychotherapy – not that that was much help for women with sexual problems, given the ignorant and misguided ideas about female sexuality held by most psychiatrists and psychoanalysts at the time.

Life was even more difficult if you were gay. Kinsey's sexual orientation findings – that many 'normal' people were neither exclusively gay nor exclusively heterosexual – were largely ignored. Psychoanalysts were trained to treat homosexuality as a perversion. Aversion therapy and chemical castration were common treatments. Homosexuality was also a crime. Alan Turing, who is now celebrated for inventing the first computer – just in time to crack the intercepted coded messages that enabled the Allies to defeat the Nazis and helped to win the Second World War – was prosecuted in 1952 for homosexual acts. The judge gave him a horrible choice: chemical castration or prison. He chose chemical castration but committed suicide two years later.

Such moral puritanism wasn't only aimed at women and gays. Married men may have had considerably more power, but even for them there was a downside. Many men, like my father, had experienced trauma in the recent war, but they had no language to talk about their feelings. As fathers, they were expected to be strong and stoic. They were largely absent from the family home all day. They were emotionally isolated by their role as providers and protectors. And in the bedroom, they felt under pressure to 'perform like a man', where any sexual activities other than the missionary position were disapproved of.

As late as 1960, Penguin Books were tried under the Obscene Publications Act for publishing the full unexpurgated version of *Lady Chatterley's Lover* by D. H. Lawrence. The novel had been declared obscene as long ago as 1928 because of its explicit descriptions of sex. In fact, the novel is a complex psychological portrayal of three lonely and unhappy people. Lady Chatterley's wheelchair-bound husband has been left bitter and impotent because of his severe injuries in the First World War. Lady Chatterley, still a young woman, finds herself isolated, childless and sexually frustrated. The gamekeeper who becomes her lover – also a traumatised war veteran – is estranged from his wife and living a lonely, sexless life in a cabin in the woods. But the moral outrage about the novel ignored the very difficult life circumstances each of these three characters were facing. Instead it focussed obsessively on Lawrence's vivid portrayals of sex: an upper-class, married woman enjoying outdoor sex in woodland glades with a lover who was also married – and possibly even worse, he was from a lower class. If we switch the genders and imagine the novel was about an upper-class married man enjoying outdoor sex with a servant girl, or even raping her, the novel would barely have received a mention in the popular press. However, this was 1960. Times were changing. Penguin Books won the case and the landmark ruling was said to usher in the so-called sexual revolution.

The 1960s was also the decade when the sexologists William Masters and Virginia Johnson hit the headlines. The aim of their research was to study the orgasm itself. This involved detailed observations and scientific measurements of volunteers, men and women, having intercourse in their laboratory. Many of the women, recruits from a local brothel, were also asked to masturbate using an alarming looking dildo, affectionately known as

Ulysses. This seems odd to me, as Kinsey had already established that most women who masturbated didn't use dildos or any form of vaginal penetration. But sadly, Masters and Johnson had decided that women who did not orgasm during penetration had a condition they labelled 'coital orgasmic inadequacy'. As a result, they excluded these women from their laboratory research.

Oh dear! This seems suspiciously close to the old Freudian notion that women who do not orgasm during penetration, by a man or by Ulysses, were sexually immature or inadequate. However, despite this disservice to womankind, the results of their research supported Kinsey's findings: there is only one kind of female orgasm, not two, and all female orgasms are clitoral. The orgasm experienced during intercourse is caused by indirect clitoral stimulation. Their attempt to explain this puzzling contradiction simply added to the confusion: 'Sociocultural influence more often than not places woman in a position in which she must adapt, sublimate, inhibit, or even distort her natural capacity to function sexually in order to fulfil her genetically assigned role (i.e., breeding). Herein lies a major source of woman's sexual dysfunction.'

They also discovered that, at a purely physiological level, the orgasm experienced by both men and women when masturbating was felt more acutely than when they had sexual intercourse. But this little gem was slightly lost amid the controversy about the myth of the vaginal orgasm and criticism of their research methods.

At last women are talking about sex, at least to each other

In the 1970s, the sexologist Shere Hite joined the debate. In Hite's opinion, by giving women the impression that not having an orgasm during intercourse was sick or abnormal, Masters and Johnson were perpetuating the usual patriarchal attitudes towards women in their research. She was determined to redress the balance. Following in Kinsey's footsteps, Hite's research also took the form of questionnaires. Her aim was to listen to what women themselves were saying about their most intimate sexual feelings. Three thousand women aged 14 to 78 responded, and in 1976 the results were published in *The Hite Report, A Nationwide Study of Female Sexuality*.

Hite dared to think outside the usual male-centric box:

> To assume that intercourse is the basic expression of female sexuality, during which the woman should orgasm, and then to analyse women's 'responses' to intercourse is to look at the issue backwards. What should be done is to look at what women are actually experiencing, what they enjoy and when they orgasm and then draw conclusions.

She began by tackling the taboo subject of female masturbation and made what was at the time a startling assertion; rather than masturbation being an indication of sexual immaturity it provides the key to understanding female sexuality.

Her study found that 82 percent of women experienced orgasm naturally through masturbation, and some from a very early age, so long as their parents didn't stop them by telling them it was dirty or wicked. She hailed this as a cause for celebration precisely because masturbation is such an easy source of orgasm for most women.

But many of the women who answered her questionnaire weren't celebrating. Whilst most of the women said they enjoyed the physical release, many of them remained very ambivalent. The various words they used to describe this feeling were lonely, guilty, unwanted, sad, selfish, silly, bad, ashamed, uncomfortable about themselves, adrift, pathetic, empty, cheap, dirty, self-conscious and even disgusted with themselves.

This complex mixture of shame and confusion about masturbation was exacerbated by another of Hite's findings: over 70 percent of women, the majority, found it difficult or impossible to orgasm during intercourse alone. The women's feelings about this make sad reading: 'A woman who has an orgasm is more of a woman, a real woman.' 'I feel judged, and also judge myself when I don't have an orgasm.' 'I still feel a constant need to know if I am normal sexually. And I still feel inadequate or immature that

I require manual stimulation to reach an orgasm.' 'I am especially shy when I have sex with new partners because I am ashamed I don't have orgasms during intercourse.' In other words, they thought they weren't normal sexually; they must be inadequate and immature if they needed oral or manual stimulation. They blamed themselves; something was wrong with them, they must have a mental block or a problem relaxing and letting themselves go. Or, they hadn't yet met 'Mr Right'.

Hite's conclusion was different. She realised that if 70 percent of women did not reach orgasm during intercourse, 'What we thought was an individual problem is neither unusual nor a problem.' The simple fact is that the penis thrusting in the vagina does not give most women the kind of physical stimulation of the clitoris they require to orgasm. This is hardly surprising given that, as Kinsey and Masters and Johnson had already established, all female orgasms are a result of direct or indirect clitoral stimulation and, like the male orgasm, follow the same physiological pattern. Presumably the 30 percent of women who said they experienced orgasms during intercourse were physiologically enabled to reach a clitoral orgasm in this way.

But the issue of perception is also important. Some women said when they masturbated they reached orgasm more quickly and their orgasm was more intense. Their experience of the orgasm during penetration was more complex. They described feelings of intense excitement followed by satisfaction, but they were not entirely sure whether they had come. As one woman put it: 'My masturbation orgasm is very intense. . . . But there have been many times in sex with a man when I have been very excited, and I have felt a rise and somewhat of a plateau and satisfied after. Then I wonder, "did I come or didn't I?" and I honestly don't know, because I didn't feel the explosive charge and super-release. I think orgasms vary in intensity, so I sometimes think maybe I had a little one. But it frustrates me when I don't know for sure'.

Another woman said: 'Clitoral orgasm gives me a full-blown climax. During intercourse, none of the flash sensations occur, but there is a tremendous calm and loving feeling that makes me cry – kind of like having an emotional (rather than physical) orgasm'.

There appears, from some of the women's accounts of their experience of 'vaginal orgasm', to be a strong psychological component. Whilst the orgasm may be less physically intense than that achieved from clitoral stimulation it was more emotionally satisfying because of the satisfaction gained from intimacy. As one woman put it: 'with penetration I feel more whole and more loved'. And 'masturbation is lonely'. But Hite's concern was that some women who think they are having orgasms during intercourse may not be. Instead they were describing plateaus of intense feeling. She worried that women may feel pressured to use 'emotional orgasms' as a substitute for the real thing.

Why do women fake it?

Things haven't changed much for many 21st-century couples. The most common sexual intercourse sequence – foreplay, penetration and thrusting until the man reaches his orgasm – is still mainly about the man's needs. Most men will engage in a little manual and oral stimulation, but they still expect the women to reach orgasm during intercourse. And the problem for many women is that they are still too ashamed and embarrassed to communicate their needs to their partners. As women who responded to Hite's questionnaire all those years ago put it: 'I kind of hate to ask my man for things, for fear of being a bother.' 'I feel guilty, selfish, uncomfortable, if my partner doesn't quite know what he is doing.' 'I would not ask him [to masturbate me] . . . He feels this is a reflection on his sexual abilities, i.e., his penis should do the job. I couldn't tell him that his penis could not possibly do the job as well.' 'It was the holy writ for me not to make a man feel inadequate and to suggest that he do something more or different would have been to appear to suggest he was inadequate.' 'Because they didn't have any idea what to do with the clitoris and I hate to give an anatomy lecture in the middle of love-making.'

In other words, many women were – and I believe still are – more concerned with looking after their man's ego than to attending to their own sexual needs. As one woman put it: she faked it to dispel his anxiety. If he keeps asking, 'have you come yet? I just said yes.

Sometimes he would even tell me how many times I came, and I didn't have the heart to tell him I hadn't come at all.'

By faking, she is reassuring him about his sexual performance and making him feel good about his manhood. This may not give her sexual fulfilment, but her ability to give him pleasure makes her feel good as a woman in another way.

The women in Hite's report gave a variety of reasons for faking it, such as 'If I really like a man I want him to think I enjoyed it more than I did.' 'If I think he's getting bored, impatient, disappointed in me.' 'Because I thought it was the only way he would continue to want me.' There's an air of desperation about statements like these. They feel that they must have an orgasm, otherwise the man will think they are not as sexy as other women. They are convinced that men enjoy making love more to women who have orgasms, and if they don't have an orgasm the man will feel bad, lose interest and even leave her. This is typical of that old pernicious fear so many women have of being compared to other women who might look better and do it better, and ultimately the fear of being abandoned and replaced by a woman who appears to be more easily satisfied – or fakes it better!

The biggest concern for many women was, and still is, how they appear in their man's eyes. Top of the list is their physical appearance, they want to look beautiful. But women also learn early in life that to be desirable to men is to be seen to desire what men like to see women desiring. Nowadays, many girls find out how men like to see women enjoying sex through Internet pornography. Female porn stars are the ultimate divas when it comes to faking orgasms. The problem is that using female porn stars as role models for how to do sex exacerbates the apparently impossible conflict between what a woman really needs for her own sexual satisfaction and her need to be desirable to men. By faking it, she is demonstrating that it is more important that her boyfriend or husband sees her having an orgasm than that she is satisfying herself by having an orgasm; it is more important that she appears sexy to him than to tune into the sensations she is really experiencing in her own body. By faking it, she can appear to be everything he could possibly want in a woman – his unselfish nurturing mother *and* his ideal sex goddess. If she doesn't have an orgasm, at least she has the consolation prize of enjoying her sexual power over him.

As one of my clients put it, she feels confident and sexy when she's acting the part, performing the sexy moves like she's seen women do in porn videos, because she believes she looks good in his eyes and she knows what to do to make him excited. But the idea of suggesting that he stimulates her clitoris to give her an orgasm, or showing him how to do it, is just too embarrassing. She loves playing with his penis to give him an orgasm, she finds this very exciting and it turns her on. She likes the power she has when she does this; she likes the feeling of being in control. But she couldn't imagine him doing the same for her. She would look ugly for a start. And she was sure she wouldn't know how to 'let go', although she wasn't sure what she would have to let go of. She thought maybe it was something to do with the fact that she hates feeling vulnerable and losing control.

But problems inevitably arise if a woman fakes it for too long. It may be satisfying enough in the early romantic stages of a love affair, but what happens when the idealisation, mutual admiration, falling-in-love phase of the relationship begins to wear a little thin? What happens when she finally admits, at least to herself, that she is left frustrated by their lovemaking? She's been slipping away to the bathroom after sex to masturbate in secret. She wants to share her orgasm with him, but she's been faking it for so long – how does she find the courage to tell him the truth and show him what she really needs him to do to enable her to have a real orgasm? For many women, this transition can be difficult or impossible to face.

So once again we find the same old issue: how the most important thing for many women is how she appears in men's eyes. She cannot risk being merely wholeheartedly herself in the moment, unself-conscious and unashamed. Instead she is split in two: she is both as she feels herself to be in the moment and at the same time another part of her is viewing herself critically, judging her physical appearance and her performance as a woman as if through the eyes of a male beholder. This doesn't mean she's not gaining pleasure, it's just that her pleasure is psychological. It's about her power – if you make a man feel like a 'real man', then you feel like a 'real woman'. And it's about her security – if you appear to be giving him what you think he wants, he won't abandon you.

Is the relationship more important for women?

Eighty-seven percent of women who answered Hite's questionnaire answered 'Yes' to the question: 'Do you enjoy sexual intercourse?' This was irrespective of whether they had an orgasm during intercourse or not. In other words, for these women the overall quality of the sexual relationship was more important to them than having an orgasm. What they valued most was the expression of love, affection, intimacy and closeness. During intercourse they felt loved, happy, secure, fulfilled, needed and sometimes a sense of euphoria. They felt successful, competent, beautiful, and adored. They liked men, they loved men's bodies and they enjoyed the pleasure they were able to give to men: 'I feel a sense of euphoria – I am successful, competent and beautiful.' 'It makes me feel important and wanted.' 'I am fulfilling the reason for my womanly existence.' 'I feel renewed as a woman.'

These intense feelings of well-being would also explain what Hite called the 'vaginal ache' – an intense desire experienced by many women to be penetrated or filled by their man. As one woman put it: 'I feel an urgent yearning way deep inside to envelop and take him inside me.' In other words, women may need clitoral stimulation to orgasm, but for many women deep penetration is an equally vital part of their sexual pleasure. Women desire and need both.

What shouts out from the clamour of women's voices that fill the pages of *The Hite Report* is that what gives women the most satisfaction during lovemaking is far more varied and subtler than the old stereotype of the man thrusting to orgasm. Yet, sadly, in our modern world of ubiquitous Internet porn and the easy availability of sexual partners through apps like Tinder, little has changed. Too many men still expect the woman to reach orgasm during penetration, and too many women are still too embarrassed or ashamed to talk to their sexual partner about what they really need.

There's an old joke: women fake orgasms to have relationships, while men fake relationships to have orgasms. I think it's more of a bitter irony than a joke. But what's really going on with men beneath the bravado?

Men talk about their sexual anxiety

The Hite Report on Male Sexuality was first published in 1981. Hite used the same method for the men's version – a questionnaire with the aim of listening to what men themselves were saying about their experience of sex and their most intimate sexual feelings. What comes up repeatedly in the survey are the connections between the man's feelings about his ability to perform, the pressure he feels to give women an orgasm, and his sense of himself as a 'real man'. The most common worries men have about sex are whether they will get hard at the appropriate moment; whether their penis and their erection are big enough; and whether they will be able to keep going for long enough before ejaculation.

Even though Hite published her report almost 40 years ago, performance anxiety and the pressure many men feel to perform sex like a 'traditional man' or a porn star is a theme that frequently comes up in psychotherapy sessions with my male clients. George's story is a typical example.

George, a journalist in his mid-thirties, told me he could not shake off the feeling that he had to give his girlfriend a vaginal orgasm, even though his girlfriend had told him that she needed clitoral stimulation to orgasm. On the face of it, he knew this was absurd. He knew about female sexuality, he had even read the *Hite Report*, or at least dipped into it enough to know the mythical vaginal orgasm didn't exist. But myths in our highly sexualised society about the imperative for men to perform sexually in the traditional stereotypically masculine manner remain so ingrained that they are very difficult to shift.

For George, 'normal sex' in a loving relationship came with a caveat: he believed that his job as the man was to please his girlfriend. This made him anxious about ejaculating too quickly, even though he knew his girlfriend's pleasure was not entirely dependent on penetration and the length of time he took to reach his orgasm. George's particularly intense need to please his girlfriend, and the anxiety he experienced about being a disappointment to her, may have had some psychological roots in a feeling that he had been a disappointment to his mother. This was a theme that frequently arose in his therapy, particularly when it emerged that George had projected his fear of being a disappointment to his mother onto me. But before we resort to psychoanalytic theories, it is important to remember that anxiety about disappointing the woman during sex by ejaculating too soon is one of the most common causes of sexual anxiety in men. As George himself had realised, when it came to sex his feelings weren't entirely rational. He was educated, he had read all the right books, yet he still felt his manhood was somehow at stake when it came to his sexual performance.

Like George, many men who answered Hite's questionnaire said they suffered from performance anxiety. One man crossly described his feelings as: 'the immense pressure to 1) get an erection, 2) keep the erection, 3) thrust exactly the way my partner likes it (with no help from her telling me how she likes it), 4) last longer than ten to fifteen minutes without prematurely ejaculating, and 5) thrust without hurting my partner when I do ejaculate – [it] is just too much to do it right each and every time.'

For some men the perplexing issue was just not knowing if, and when, their partner wanted sex. One man put it this way: 'I feel like, what does she want? If I'm not sure I can get it up right then, I sometimes think it might be nice to lay around together, but usually I decide that I had better act cold and say no because I don't know what she wants. . . . I don't like feeling called upon to respond as a male . . . you know (grunt, grunt) me man, you woman, I fuck you – etc.' Sadly, his defence against his fear of not being able to get an erection on demand to prove his manhood is acting cold (i.e. shutting the woman out). I can't count the amount of times I have heard women say how unhappy they are because their partner seems to have gone cold and is shutting them out. If only their partner would talk to them and tell them what is going on! They may also like to just 'lay around together' and see what happens.

One of the big concerns expressed by men was whether the woman had an orgasm or not. If she didn't orgasm, was it his fault? For instance, in response to Hite's question about post-coital thoughts, one man wrote: '1) did she come and if not, should I feel responsible? 2) Fear of obligation. Now that we have had sex this is more serious. 3) Disappointment when a sexual exchange still leaves me and my partner far from true intimacy.' Many men said they felt guilty and self-critical after their 'performance'. Some even said they felt depressed after sex; they worried that their 'performance' wasn't good enough: 'Sometimes I get depressed and have feelings of failure and self-hatred. It should have been longer, bigger, better, etc.'

Another man said he felt guilty because he had satisfied himself: 'There seems to be a stigma now for men to be super-cocks – continue, continue, do for the woman. I love giving – yet I must do for me. I know I am being defensive, probably against an unseen enemy, yet the pressure is there.' It's not difficult to sense the anger behind his words, particularly when he raises the spectre of an unseen enemy. But what is this unseen enemy? I think it is partly the misguided belief many men have that they must keep thrusting for as long as possible to satisfy the woman and the guilt they feel when they give in to their own orgasm. The guilt generates a feeling of defensiveness and an impulse to blame the demanding woman for causing the pressure rather than entertaining the idea that it might all be in his head. I think what this man is really expressing is a problem in all intimate sexual relationships irrespective of gender. The big question is:

> how can we be sensitive to the other's needs and satisfy our own needs at the same time?

Thirty-nine percent of men in Hite's survey said they had had trouble having an erection at some time or other, and the fear of it happening, or not happening when required, was always present.

One man said: 'It is very embarrassing when it happens. I was relieved to discover from a woman friend that it is not a problem unique to me. But the pressure is still on men to perform. Men are horny, lustful beasts, why aren't you tearing at me with your giant erection? It's a myth, but still one that haunts us from over our shoulders'. Another man described the shock of inexplicably losing his erection during intercourse as: 'What the hell happened? … How delicately am I balanced, anyway? It is frustrating and embarrassing. It makes me feel like I am a little helpless boy, guilty usually. I feel ashamed.' I think the sentiments expressed by this man are sad and incredibly telling. Men are far more delicately balanced than they realise or are prepared to admit.

According to the *Guardian* newspaper, a recent study of 2,000 British men found that 50 percent of men in their thirties reported difficulties in getting and maintaining an erection ('Why Do So Many Young Men Have Performance Anxiety?' *Guardian* 2018). If anything, the social pressure on young men to be perfect sexual performers has become even greater.

> I have been treating men for thirty years and there's no doubt that we are seeing more young men today than we used to. Often these are men who appear to be super-healthy: they are slim, they exercise, they're young, and you think, 'Why on earth have these men got sexual difficulties?'
>
> Dr Douglas Savage, Centre for Men's Health

Internet pornography and social media are exacerbating the problem. As one of the men in the *Guardian* article said: 'What if my girlfriend is telling her friends?' He was also worried 'about the possibility of his shame going viral online. "If it gets on social media you are screwed"'.

Adam, an attractive man in his mid-twenties, came to see me for therapy because he was anxious and depressed. It soon emerged that he had split up from his long-term girlfriend and he was in despair by what he described as his 'pathetic attempts to find girls on Tinder.' About an hour after he met the first girl, they went to her place to have sex. But as he put it, 'I couldn't get it up'. He was devastated, convinced he was 'inadequate, a failure because he couldn't do casual sex like other guys.' He had continued to go on

Tinder and even arranged to meet other girls, but each time he 'went into panic mode and cancelled.' It was as if the humiliation and shame he had experienced by his one failure to get an erection was stuck inside him like a trauma. He was reassured when I said that it wasn't so unusual for men to have trouble getting an erection on a first date or when they were anxious. But when I suggested that maybe it would help if he got to know the girl a little first, he said I was being old-fashioned; girls expect sex on the first date.

Several men who responded to Hite's questionnaire said that they felt incredibly relieved when they realised that they weren't alone, that it wasn't unusual for men to be unable to get an erection or to lose their erection. Nevertheless, the fear of it happening and the embarrassment and shame remained. On the other hand, a few men pointed out that sex can be enjoyable without an erection and in any case, erections can come and go during sex. But the problem remains. If you worry about not getting an erection at the right moment, then you are less likely to. Anxiety itself can bring about the feared result. Unlike women who can use lubricants and fake their sexual excitement, men can't fake an erection; they can't will an erection into being, and if an erection does not materialise when wanted, they can feel utterly inadequate as a man. The effect on their partner can also be devastating if the woman assumes that the problem is her fault; she is just not attractive enough or he doesn't love her enough. But one man reported that he had discovered a great cure: 'being open with my lover and telling her how frightened I was of failing, etc. So, we slept together for about a week, just cuddling, without any pressure on me to get an erection, and by and by nature took its course'. In other words, 'the cure' he had discovered was talking to each other about sexual feelings. What an excellent idea!

Men are just as confused about premature ejaculation. Some men think it means ejaculating just before or immediately after penetration. Other men interpret it as the man not being able to keep going for long enough, or not being able to delay their ejaculation until the woman reaches her orgasm. Seventy-four percent of men in Hite's survey expressed concern about whether they kept going for long enough. And most men thought this was the main reason why women failed to reach an orgasm during intercourse. One man said he considered ejaculating too soon as a failed test of virility. Another man described it as showing 'a lack of self-control. I don't like it because it's worse than nothing for a woman. Plus, it's embarrassing.' Quite a few men talked about how they tried to control themselves to keep going for longer; how they would attempt to dampen their excitement by thinking unexciting thoughts. But apart from the fact that deliberately thinking about something excessively dull whilst having great sex is counterintuitive, it didn't work very well either.

A few men blamed their penis size. They thought their partner couldn't orgasm because their penis was too small. Most men said they wished their penis was bigger. Men also compared themselves unfavourably to the men in porn videos. They marvelled at the studs' penis size and staying power: 'They were hard as rock and lasted two or three women!' How could those porn studs stay hard for so long and just keep on going? The men (and it is usually men) who make money from pornographic videos, are of course using all the tricks of the filmmakers' trade – camera angles, extreme close-ups, editing together many days' filming into one ten-minute video – to create a believable illusion of reality to stimulate their customers' voyeuristic desires. Tragically, the easy accessibility of all this fake sex on tablets and mobile phones has become one of the main ways young boys imagine they are learning how to do sex.

When Hite asked men about whether they felt a pressure to satisfy the woman she discovered that the majority realised that women often did not orgasm during intercourse. And yet even this was experienced as another source of pressure. Many men still felt it was their fault. Some even mentioned feeling 'threatened, not sensitive enough, I did not do it right', or 'I was in too much of a selfish rush to get my rocks off.' What was increasingly apparent from most of the men's responses was the pressure they felt to satisfy the woman by thrusting during intercourse. Quite a few men expressed their frustration and even anger with women for thinking that a good lover should be able to make the woman orgasm without even telling them how, or what she wants.

As one man put it: 'If they would only tell me how, I would do my damnedest to make sure that they reached orgasm.' Another man said: 'I feel shame, remorse, guilt, not a man, and I hate her for making me feel that way.' Another man blamed his pent-up emotions on his wife as well as himself: 'Then there is sex immediately in front of you and I get uncontrollably excited and go off. Does it bother me? Yes, it makes me hate myself and my wife just that much more. It makes me feel inadequate and unmanly not satisfying myself or my wife'. In other words, the psychological damage to their relationship, of not talking to each other about sex and learning to understand what's going on for each other, was having a hugely detrimental effect on their marriage.

But some men persisted in blaming the woman if she didn't orgasm during intercourse like a 'normal woman' should. They said things like: 'My first thought is that she is or has become frigid.' Or 'I would question my performance.... But I would also question her state of mind. I wouldn't question my masculinity.' Or 'It's her fault. I am man enough.'

The tragedy of the myth of the vaginal orgasm, for men as well as women, is that it impacts negatively on both sexes. If men are afraid they may not be able to keep going for long enough to satisfy the woman, or they may lose their erection trying, they feel themselves to be in a vulnerable position. For some men this anxiety about their vulnerability is experienced as a fundamental threat to their manhood. The only way they can avoid unbearable feelings of vulnerability is by overt displays of masculine dominance and cutting short displays of physical affection and foreplay and getting on with the 'real business'; penetration and their own orgasm.

Many women sense their partner's anxiety and, to reassure him of his masculinity, fake orgasms. This may make their man feel good about himself, but it often leaves women feeling frustrated and even causes some women to lose interest in sex altogether.

The good news is that there were men who answered Hite's questionnaire who knew their partner's satisfaction depended on clitoral stimulation. Acting on this had improved their love making. One man said: 'Manually stimulating the clitoris during intercourse used to strike me as unnatural, but now I recognise the need and even enjoy it.' These men said they had discovered that their sexual relationships were far more mutually rewarding and more fun: 'to take turns being "selfish" . . . making love in the masculine way and, later, on another day, in a feminine way.'

But the questions remain; why is there, apparently, a 'masculine way' and a 'feminine way'? Why is it that the men and women don't fit sexually?

The genders don't fit: Is this a design fault or a trick of evolution?

Evolutionary psychology and neuroscience are fashionable areas of research in the 21st century and they have both addressed the perplexing question of the female orgasm. In 2005 the *New Scientist* came up with a provocative headline: 'Genes Blamed for the Fickle Female Orgasm'. This was a piece about a British study into women's ability to climax – or not. But underlying the fun headline was the same old question: how come women don't orgasm in their vaginas as they should? Surely it would vastly improve sex for both genders.

The leaders of this survey concluded that the answer lies in evolution and the genes. If women reached orgasm too easily, they wouldn't be very good selectors. The survival of the species requires more than brawn – the strongest male with the biggest weapon gets the female – it needs brains and the ability to be good nurturers and providers. The genes of women who were satisfied too easily were selected out over time, and the fussy women who wanted the brightest and most intelligent men in the cave survived. In other words, we are back to Masters and Johnson's assertion that woman's primary function isn't her own sexual pleasure: 'she must adapt, sublimate, inhibit, or even distort her natural capacity to function sexually in order to fulfil her genetically assigned role (i.e., breeding)'.

Elizabeth Lloyd, an American scientist who also looked to evolution for the answer takes this idea a step further. In *The Case of the Female Orgasm* (2005), she points out that the reason for the male orgasm is obvious: it makes men eager for sex, without which the species would die out. But the female orgasm isn't necessary for reproductive success. The females of most animal species don't have orgasms. (How does she know?) Whatever, for Lloyd, the pertinent question is not why do so many women have problems reaching an orgasm, but why do women have orgasms at all? Lloyd's theory is that the female orgasm is an evolutionary by-product of the male orgasm, just as the clitoris is a biological remnant of the penis. This seems to be at odds with Kinsey's finding that the area of tactile sensitivity is greater in the female genital area. It also doesn't explain why many women feel their sexual needs just as strongly as many men. Their problem isn't their lack of sexual desire; it's their lack of sexual fulfilment in a cultural climate that even today places women's sexual needs as lesser than the needs of men.

Where do we go from here?

Despite the findings of the sexologists over many decades, and the fact that 21st-century culture appears to be more obsessed with sex than ever, many women are still too ashamed, too self-conscious or too afraid to talk frankly about their sexual needs with their partner. They still habitually satisfy men's needs rather than their own. Many men are still preoccupied with their performance and their 'manhood' being on display.

As each new generation of women begins to understand their bodies and to pay attention to their own sexual fulfilment, their anxiety, about the effect this may have on men and threaten their relationships, becomes so great women promptly repress their own sexual needs. It's as if, when it comes to the truth about female sexuality, there are periods of sexual enlightenment followed by periods of forgetting what has been learnt, or sexual mass amnesia. This may also be a symptom of the regular backlashes against feminism that take place every few decades. It wasn't that my mother didn't know about Kinsey's findings; after she died I came across a dusty old copy of Kinsey's *Sexual Behaviour in the Human Female* amongst her books. It's just that in the hyper-conservative climate of the 1950s, she found it too difficult or too disturbing to talk to her husband or her children or anyone else about what she knew.

Whatever the evolutionary or genetic reasons for the apparently 'bad fit' between men and women, there has certainly been a psychological impact on both sexes. The penis is undoubtedly bigger than the clitoris. But whilst the clitoris is safely hidden away, the penis – whether it is flaccid or erect – is on display, which risks the man feeling vulnerable. I think the excessive male concern with size, performance and masculinity is a defence against this ever-present fear of their sexual vulnerability. Consciously or unconsciously, women are aware of man's vulnerability, which may explain their excessive concern with looking after their man's ego when on the surface it appears that the male ego is quite good at looking after itself.

It would help if the two *Hite Reports* were included as an essential part of sex and relationship studies in schools. This would debunk the many myths about sex and give young people an opportunity to learn to talk authentically about sex and sexual problems. It would also help if more adults were able to talk to each other about sex in the bedroom, or wherever they have sex. But when it comes to the psychological complexity of what is going on in our sexual relationships, talking honestly about sex is only part of the story.

3 What have parents got to do with our sexual relationships?

On love, sexual rivalry and Oedipus

Fathers and mothers have an insidious way of turning up in places where we think they don't belong, such as our sexual relationships. This is not so surprising. Our parents are our first role models and our first love objects. How they love us, or withhold their love, or are incapable to loving, will affect our ability to love and be loved in later life, and even the kind of partner we find or whether we find a partner at all. Conversations about parents are one of the most fruitful topics to arise in the consulting room even if, as far as the client is concerned, the reason they have come to therapy has nothing to do with their parents.

I try not to mention the Oedipus complex when I am talking to clients. I don't want to risk the 'Who the hell was Oedipus and what is a complex anyway?' reaction. Or 'I thought she was a nice modern psychotherapist; surely Freud died out with the dinosaurs!' It's fashionable in these days of 'evidence-based psychology' to dismiss Freud. Some readers may also be surprised that I haven't ditched Freud, given the damage caused by his mistaken ideas about female sexuality, not to mention the suffering of gay people who were told by Freudian analysts that their sexuality was an unnatural perversion. However, love him or loathe him, it was Freud who made the great breakthrough when he discovered the significance of the unconscious mind when searching for a deeper understanding of sex and gender and what makes us who we are.

Part of the problem with the Oedipus complex is the language. People panic when they hear the label, assuming it must mean something is awfully wrong with them. They don't realise that a 'complex', according to my dictionary, is merely 'a group of emotional impulses that have been banished from the conscious mind but continue to influence a person's behaviour'. 'Emotional impulses' is a horrible phrase. I prefer to think of a swirling mass of powerful emotions, such as love, joy, desire, rivalry, envy, guilt and rage – emotions we all experienced in childhood in response to our parents or care-givers and even siblings, that continue to influence our adult behaviour. If we remind ourselves of its proper meaning, there is not a person on the planet who doesn't have a complex. But why did Freud choose to name the Oedipus complex after the hero of an ancient Greek tragedy? Can the tragic events that befell Oedipus really help us to understand ourselves in the modern world?

Some readers may know the story of Oedipus, but here is a quick reminder. Once upon a time in a royal palace, baby Oedipus was born. Soon after the birth, the Oracle issued a chilling prophecy: when baby Oedipus grew up, he would murder his father and marry his mother. Oedipus's father, the king, was horrified and ordered his servant to have the baby killed. Oedipus's mother, the queen, abandoned her baby to its fate. The servant took the baby to a remote mountainside and left it there to die. But Oedipus did not die; he was rescued by a passing shepherd and brought up in a neighbouring kingdom. Many years later when Oedipus reached manhood, he returned to the kingdom of his birth. He met a man on the road, they got into a fight and Oedipus killed him, not knowing this man was his real father. Later he married the wife of the man he had killed, not knowing she was in fact his real mother. When Oedipus learned the awful truth, he flew into a terrible rage and ordered his servant to bring him a sword to cut out the womb of the woman he now knew was both his wife and his mother. But his wife/mother had heard that Oedipus had discovered the truth and already hanged herself. Oedipus cut her body down, pulled out the pins of her dress and used the pins to gouge out his own eyes.

No wonder poor Oedipus resorted to extreme self-harm. What could be more traumatising for any young man than to discover he has unwittingly committed patricide and had sex with his own mother?

To explain why he had chosen to name his complex after Oedipus, Freud wrote:

> It is the fate of us all, perhaps, to direct our first sexual impulse towards our mother and our first hatred and our first murderous wish against our father. Our dreams convince us this is so.

Freud also made this devastating statement:

> His [Oedipus's] destiny moves us only because it might have been ours – because the Oracle laid the same curse on us before our birth as upon him.
>
> (Freud 1899)

Freud never missed a beat when he saw an opportunity for dramatic effect. But what have murderous impulses and incestuous desires got to do with the fate of us all?

For all babies, their mother or primary care-giver is the centre of their emotional universe, she is the primary object of their nurture, love, rage and hate (see Chapter 9). Gradually, as the baby grows it develops an awareness of its own identity separate from its mother. The little boy realises he is male, like his father. The little girl realises that she is the same gender as her mother and different from her father. With this dawning awareness of gender differences, the boy's story and the girl's story begin to diverge. I will begin by talking about the boy's story and save the girl's story for later.

The boy's story

So, how does this very early stage in the little boy's life relate to the Oedipus story? Freud believed that as the little boy becomes increasingly absorbed with the primitive sexual sensations in his body and his growing awareness of his gender as a boy, he becomes increasingly curious about his mother's female body. He begins to nurture secret desires and fantasies about his mother. He wishes he could have her all to himself, but he is also afraid that if his father, who is his main rival for his mother's body, finds out about his fantasies – that he wants Daddy out of the way, so he can marry Mummy – his father may punish him by castrating him, which is a most dire image of being de-sexed or emasculated. I don't think it's helpful to think of these desires or fantasies as incestuous, murderous or even particularly sexual. That would be to assume that Freud was taking the Oedipus story literally, rather than seeing it as a pathway to an understanding of our unconscious minds. Freud himself referred to these childish bodily sensations and impulses as driven by a 'damped down libido'.

In short, the Oedipus complex refers to the boy's transition from his primitive identification as a baby with his mother, to his realisation that he is a boy and he should be identifying with his father. Freud thought the gender identification with father by around about the age of four or five was a sign of the successful completion of the Oedipal stage in a boy's sexual development. It was this notion of a so-called successful Oedipal transition which, sadly, contributed to the now rightly discredited idea that homosexuality is caused by an unsuccessful or incomplete Oedipal phase of development. However, irrespective of whether men are straight or gay, complicated feelings of competition and rivalry, as well as love and affection, remain a prominent feature in relations between fathers and sons, certainly for the rest of childhood and adolescence and often throughout adult life.

The Oedipus complex has been a subject of controversy ever since Freud first formulated his theory. Part of the problem, as we saw in Chapter 1, is the reluctance to think about children as having sexual feelings, let alone that they can also feel consumed by sexual desires, rivalries and murderous fantasies towards parents. This is, perhaps, an understandable resistance to the stirring up of primitive emotions that Freud believed were so disturbing we long ago repressed them in our unconscious. However, the first love we experienced with our mothers and fathers, and whatever individual peculiarities characterised this love, which nowadays is more usually referred to as the Oedipal triangle, typically remain the source of the feelings and projections that arise in our later love relationships. (As we will see in Chapter 5, attachment theory research backs this up.)

The idea that little boys might nurture fantasies of wanting to marry their mother is just too much for our modern, scientific sensibility. The fact that very small boys frequently declare that they want to marry mummy is amusing rather than reflecting anything deeper. By the time boys have grown up to be men, the imaginative world they inhabited as a child is often long forgotten. Few men readily recall that their mother ever featured in their sexual fantasies. Whilst literal depictions of sex and violence and murder are a source of endless fascination in adult drama and pornography, few men care to analyse the roots of the dark sexual and violent feelings buried in their own unconscious.

However, it is not unusual for men to marry women who are like their mothers. Or they set about influencing their partner's behaviour and even their partner's physical appearance to turn her into a carbon copy of their mothers. The problem for some men is that this unconscious dynamic can numb their sexual desire for their partner, possibly because the incest taboo has kicked in. On the other hand, some men find that women who strongly resemble their mothers heightens their libidos. This was the case with one of my clients who told me he was amazed when he came across an old photo of his mother when she was young and for an instant mistook her for his wife. 'Sex with Mothers' is also on the list of most searched for phrases on Internet porn sites. This suggests that a fascination at least with the fantasy if not the reality of sex with mother is far from uncommon.

This takes me back to the gory scene in Oedipus's story when he cuts down the body of his wife/mother after she has hanged herself. The scene is macabre. But isn't it interesting that he pulls out the pins of her dress, presumably revealing the shocking sight of his wife/mother's naked body, and these are the very same pins he uses to gouge out his own eyes. I can't think of a more horrific act of self-punishment. It also tells us about his unbearable feelings when confronted with the sight of his wife/mother's naked sexuality; he blinds himself to escape from the horror of seeing the truth.

When men talk about their mothers in psychotherapy, a range of complicated and ambivalent feelings often rise to the surface. It's not unusual for the love they feel for their mothers to be accompanied by a physical awkwardness, a need to hold their mother at a distance, not to let her get too close, and a disturbing feeling of guilt that is difficult for them to understand. Men whose mothers made them husband substitutes for whatever reason – maybe because their father was seen by their mother as too weak, or their father had abandoned the family – are particularly ambivalent. Men whose mothers were too physically intimate with them when they were little, or who ignored their boundaries completely and sexually abused them, can find intimacy, or letting any woman get close, a real problem or impossible in adult life.

Men's feelings about their fathers are often just as complicated and ambivalent. Freud focussed on the fact that Oedipus killed his father to illustrate his theory that boys experience their fathers as rivals who must be got rid of, so the boy can take the father's place in his mother's affections. But what if the source of this father-son rivalry is the father, not the son? In a way, all baby boys displace the father as soon as they are born. The father looks on enviously whilst the baby eagerly sucks his mother's breast; the baby not only monopolises her body and her sexuality, he also steals her love. I think the more fathers share in the maternal role, the more these feelings of exclusion are abated. But a common problem for men I have seen in therapy has been their deeply disturbing experience of their father's 'murderous' rages towards them or their mothers. The legacy of growing up as the object of their father's rages is devastating. This is an important theme in the Oedipus drama, but one that was overlooked by Freud. The king's murderous rage was the source of the whole Oedipus drama. The king gave the order to kill his baby because he was afraid his son would grow up to murder him. In other words, the father was afraid that his son would one day depose him and take his place as king. The tragedy for Oedipus was compounded by his mother's complicity. For whatever reason, she failed to protect her baby from her murderous husband and abandoned him to his fate.

I think this is the original trauma, the Oracle's curse. It reflects a very common and deep existential fear of being abandoned, which goes hand in hand with a deep fear of dependency on a loved one and gives rise to many later problems in adult love relationships – as we shall see in Jeremy's story.

Why was Jeremy afraid of losing his virginity?

We were about 15 minutes into his first session when I asked Jeremy if he was in a relationship. It's a question I normally ask when I'm trying to get a picture of a new client's current life. But Jeremy's reaction was instant. He shot a glance at my consulting room door and for a moment I thought he was about to run out. 'I'm not here to talk about relationships,' he muttered, 'I'm here because I feel depressed, miserable and worthless.'

'That's okay, so nothing to do with relationships.' I said carefully, and I hoped, reassuringly. I could sense we were on difficult terrain.

'Well, I know it may have something to do with relationships,' he said, after a long pause. 'Actually, I think my needs are too big for any relationship. But I don't want to talk about relationships. Not yet anyway.'

I was sitting in my usual armchair on one side of the Victorian fireplace. Jeremy was seated on the sofa opposite me. He reached for the glass of water on the coffee table and took a gulp.

Jeremy was 24, a shy, serious trainee in a busy law firm. I thought he was attractive, but he said he hated his appearance. He was a little plump, but he was convinced that he was too fat, and he hated his round boyish face splattered with freckles. He had a lively smile on the occasions when he risked a smile. But for the first few sessions his manner remained tense and guarded and he often sat clutching his leg, which was balanced across one knee as if he was defending himself against me getting too close.

At first, we talked about his childhood – which was, of course, also talking about relationships, but I sensed he felt marginally safer talking about his childhood than whatever was, or was not, going on in the present. He told me he had been an over-sensitive child: 'That's what my Dad used to say about me because I used to cry a lot and he couldn't stand me crying. He used to accuse me of being a wimp, a cry baby, a miserable whinge, completely worthless, a mother's boy, not man enough. He never liked me. He doted on my sister. It was okay if she cried because she was a girl.'

His father had been a very angry man who frequently flew into furious rages with Jeremy and his mother. Jeremy was 13 when his parents split up. His sister had just left home for university. Jeremy and his mother moved to a remote house in the countryside. Changing schools and making new friends was hard. But Jeremy said he didn't mind; he preferred to spend evenings at home with his mother rather than mix with the village kids. When he had finished his homework the two of them would to curl up on the sofa together watching television with a TV dinner. 'I remember us being really happy then. But when I was 15 Mum got married again. Unbelievable! She married another angry guy who treated me and Mum like shit, just like Dad used to. I felt completely betrayed. After a while, things became so bad between me and my stepfather that I was sent away to a boys' boarding school. I think my stepfather gave Mum an ultimatum: either the boy goes, or I go. Something like that. He just wanted me out of the way. Anyway, she chose him, and I felt completely abandoned. I can't forgive her for that.'

Jeremy hated boarding school. He was too shy and unhappy to make new friends. When the other boys went out together having fun, endlessly boasting about things they had done with girls at the weekends, Jeremy buried himself in schoolwork: 'But at least I learned to stop crying. You're a dead man if you cry at boarding school. Now I never cry . . . well not with other people anyway. I think I'm all bottled up,' he said, and gave me a wry smile.

One day he arrived late for his session. He sat down and began apologising immediately: 'I'm sorry. I know you want me to come to therapy with offerings, I'm supposed to bring you feelings, but I can't because I don't feel anything. Or if I do, I can't access them when I'm here. And I'm afraid of letting you down, not being able to deliver what you want. I'm afraid I will never be able to give you what you want or expect from me. So, the therapy is pointless.'

I took a deep breath. I felt sure his fear of letting me down, and not being able to give me what he imagined I wanted, was precisely what was preventing him having an intimate relationship with anybody. I decided to risk the R word again: 'If this is how you feel about seeing me, that you are bound to let me down because you will never be able to give me what I want, then I'm wondering if this is pretty much how you feel about all close relationships?' I said.

He looked at me suspiciously: 'You mean with girls?'

I nod.

'Okay, it is pretty much how I feel, yes', he said, staring into the fireplace to avoid my eyes.

So maybe it's not your needs that are too great for a relationship to bear, it's the needs of the other person in the relationship you feel you can't meet, like you feel you can't give me what I want?

He thought about this for a while. 'Maybe, maybe it's both,' he said eventually.

I had suspected that Jeremy was still a virgin and I also had a feeling that Jeremy suspected that I knew his secret. The subject of sex was the elephant in the room. But I didn't want to push him into talking about sexual relationships because I had a feeling if I went there too soon he might leave and never come back. But each week the damn elephant was growing bigger and bigger. Until one day the elephant balloon burst.

'I've been thinking, we should be talking about relationships,' he said in a rush, as soon as he sat down for his session. 'I don't know how this happened. I'm twenty-four and I've never had a real relationship. And now it feels like it's too late. What woman would ever want a twenty-four-year-old man without . . . who has never had sex?' He glanced nervously at the door as if someone might be listening. I felt sure he had never ever told anyone this before. He rushed on with his story, his words tumbling over themselves, eager to get it over with: 'I think there's something wrong with me. I've even wondered if I was gay; the weak, crying, mother's boy thing my Dad was always on about. But I never have gay fantasies and I don't like gay porn. Also, most of my friends at work are women. They say I'm a good listener. I know it sounds stupid, but I still believe that I should be in love when I have sex – it should be 'The Relationship'.

I asked him if he had ever been in love. He said he used to be in love with a girl called Emily. They were in the same year at university and lived in the same shared house. She used to tell people he was her best friend. She often came to his room when she was lonely, and they would just hang out, talk, listen to music.

'Did you ever tell her how you felt about her?' I asked.

'I couldn't. She shared a room with her boyfriend; a super-confident, driven, macho type, into competitive sports. He was out training most evenings. She used to confide in me about what a difficult man he was. She even cried sometimes, and I would put my arm around her to comfort her. I had lots of fantasies about rescuing her.'

I was wondering if Jeremy had had fantasies of rescuing his mother from his father's rages when he was a boy. But I didn't say anything. I didn't want to interrupt his flow.

He smiled at me bitterly: 'Just before graduation she came to my room and announced she had just got engaged to macho-man. I did a pretty good job of pretending I was happy for her. She even invited me to their wedding. I went, of course. It was hell. I had wasted three miserable years at university pining for Emily in secret. Now I've left it too late, I'm trapped. How could I ever tell any girl that I am still a virgin? I suppose I could try to pretend I'm not, but I know it would show. I even tried going to a prostitute about a year ago, but I bottled out at the last minute. The thought of doing it like that disgusted me.'

He fell silent for a while before adding quietly: 'I feel ashamed all the time. I hate myself for letting this happen. I hate looking at myself in the mirror; all I can see is a hideous, pathetic, miserable, whinging wimp. It's all completely hopeless.'

'I don't think it's hopeless,' I said.

'You have to say that, don't you? It's your job. If you agree it's hopeless your client might go out there and top himself.'

'Have you thought of doing that?'

'I think about it sometimes. But I know I couldn't go through with it. I don't have the courage.'

'Jeremy, I know there are girls out there who wouldn't be put off by your lack of experience. I know, because they come to see me here, in this room. They tell me they are unhappy, lonely and what they really want is a sensitive man.'

'Maybe,' he said, without conviction.

We sat in silence for a while watching the flames of the gas fire.

Eventually, I said, 'I'm thinking about what you said you see when you look in the mirror. A pathetic, miserable, whinging wimp – isn't that what your father used to call you when you cried when you were a boy?'

'Something like that. Maybe he was right.'

'I don't think he was right. You were just a child, crying because you were scared. He sounds like a bully to me. And now you are attacking yourself with the same words he used to bully you. I'm wondering why you aren't angry with him?'

'I am, sometimes, when I'm in my flat on my own. I sometimes get into awful rages with him, with my mother, with the whole world.'

'But mostly the rage is with yourself?'

'Yes, mostly.'

After Jeremy had left the session I could almost hear his father's voice ringing in my ears: 'If you're still a virgin that just goes to prove me right; you are a worthless wimp, not man enough for any woman and certainly not man enough to be my son.' Jeremy's childhood memories of his bullying father had become his own harsh internal judge and for much of the time he felt like a worm his father had squashed under foot. No wonder he felt miserable and worthless. His father had certainly done a pretty good job of castrating him. But I also felt hopeful. Jeremy had told me about his virginity at last. The elephant was no longer in the room.

For the next few sessions we talked more about his anger with his father and his own anger. He said he hated being angry, it scared him: 'What if I have inherited my Dad's anger? I don't think I have, but the thought of being like him disgusts me.' He paused, shocked by the sudden venom in his voice. He added quietly, 'I feel guilty for saying that. He's changed now he's older, he's not so bad now. I even think he likes me a little, now I'm working in a law firm. He thinks I'm taking after him.' He gave a hollow laugh.

'Guilt can be a defence against anger.' I said. 'I think you are angry, very angry. And you've turned all that anger against yourself. That's what I hear when you tell me about your depression; you, attacking yourself.'

After he left, I had a strong feeling that he was angry with me. The following week I asked him how he felt after the last session.

'Pissed off,' he said, 'pissed off with you for trying to make me angry. Actually, I imagined myself throwing that box of tissues out of the window and smashing up your coffee table.'

'Hard table to smash, that. It's heavy.'

'I've noticed,' he said, and grinned ruefully.

'So why do you think you were so angry with me?'

'I didn't like you saying that my depression was a defence against my anger. But I've thought about it, and I think maybe you are right. And another thing that pissed me off is that you reminded me of my mother, when you said there were lots of nice, sensitive girls out there just looking for a man like me.'

'Why did that piss you off?'

'Because I'm scared, I suppose.'

'Scared of what?'

'Of messing up, of being hurt, of being rejected. I don't think I could bear that.'

'I think you could. The thing is, the only way to find a relationship is to take risks. Sometimes we are rejected, sometimes we realise the other person is not for us and we reject them. So it goes, we survive until we find the relationship that works for us.'

'You make it sound like a job application,' he grinned. 'What about falling in love?'

'Falling in love is nice, especially if you fall in love with a girl who is available.'

'You mean, not like Susan,' he smiled.

Susan was a friend at work he had said he fancied. The problem was, she was a lesbian.

After he had gone, I wondered what he was thinking about as he walked away up the street. I was thinking about the evenings he had spent as 13-year-old curled up with his mother on the sofa. Even though he said those years, when he had his mother all to himself, were 'the happy years', his mother had done him a huge disservice – she had warded off her own loneliness by turning her son into her husband substitute. This made the rejection he felt when his stepfather arrived on the scene even more painful. If he fell in love with a girl he would have to trust her, like he had once trusted his mother. What if, like his mother, the girl rejected him for another man? This might explain why the only girl he had fallen in love with at university had been unavailable, like his mother was unavailable because she belonged to a macho, manly man like his father and his stepfather. By falling in love with a girl who belonged to another man, Jeremy had unconsciously repeated the same familiar emotional dynamic formed in his childhood. His depression was his safe hiding place, his defence against ever being hurt or rejected by a woman again.

'No, I wasn't thinking about my mother,' he said, the following week when I asked him what he had been thinking about after the last session. 'I was thinking about a new girl who has just come to work in the office. Her name is Lucy. She's nice. I've been showing her the ropes.'

'You mean she's going to become your new best friend?' I was being provocative, but I couldn't resist it.'

'Maybe,' he said, 'or maybe not.'

A few weeks later he arrived for his session with a smile. We still had a lot more work to do on his trust issues. But I knew at once, something big had changed.

What about the girls?

There was an attempt to give girls an equivalent to the Oedipus complex. The psychoanalyst Carl Jung suggested the Electra complex, as if giving girls a Greek tragedy of their own like a consolation prize would solve the girl problem. But the Electra complex never really caught on because Electra's story doesn't have the same psychological resonance. We get closer to the equivalent for girls if we imagine that Oedipus was a girl. Dare we call her Oedipussy?

I find Oedipussy's story even more disturbing than that of the boy Oedipus. This could be because I am a woman. But there is something intrinsically chilling about a mother, whose primary role is to nurture and protect her new-born baby, ordering a servant to murder Oedipussy. Come to think of it, our cultural history is peppered with evil queens, wicked witches and envious stepmothers. These terrifying female characters are usually portrayed in fairy tales as cruel, jealous women who hate their daughters and stepdaughters because they are younger, more beautiful and may grow up to steal their mother's place by the king. Perhaps their fear is not so unfounded. This is precisely what Oedipussy does; she grows up and murders her mother and marries her father.

Envy and sexual rivalry between mothers and their daughters, and between women generally, has a powerful resonance deep in our psyches and in our culture generally. Oedipussy's story also gives us some insights into the sexual desires and conflicts experienced by girls and the women they are destined to become. As we saw earlier, the first object of love and rage for all babies, boys and girls is their mother or primary care-giver. But as the toddlers begin to gain a sense of their gender – that girls are the same gender as their mothers and boys as their fathers – this realisation has a profound impact on their developing sense of their own gender identity. It also changes the nature of their relationships with both their mothers and fathers. Both genders are then confronted by new and bewildering conflicts in their Oedipal triangle.

For instance, boys and girls often experience disturbing feelings of anxiety and guilt as their loyalties become split between how to please both their mother and their father. Whilst boys may take pride in identifying with their fathers and at the same time feel some anxiety about wanting their father out of the way so they can have their mother all to themselves, their mother's familiar role as their primary source of nurture and security usually remains intact. The girl faces a different conflict. If she secretly imagines herself stealing her mother's place so she can have her father all to herself, she not only feels guilty about betraying her mother's love; she also risks arousing her mother's anger and putting her hitherto secure relationship with her mother, who is also her primary love object and source of nurture, in jeopardy.

In other words, girls are caught, emotionally, between a rock and a hard place. Her father, as her new object of desire, allows her some escape from her conflicted, ambivalent feelings towards her beloved mother. But as Melanie Klein pointed out, typically girls retain some unconscious remnants of their sexual desires towards their mother's body. The girl *wants* to take her mother's place in relation to her father *and* she wants to take her father's place and have her mother's love all to herself. She wants both! This may go some way towards explaining why research into women's sexuality shows that women are more inclined than men towards bisexuality. When heterosexual women were shown images of two women having sex they often became sexually aroused. Also, many heterosexual women have sexual fantasies that involve other women, but nevertheless, in their actual sex lives they remain heterosexual. In the past this choice may have been due to fear of social disapproval, whereas nowadays more women are choosing to explore the full range of their sexual desires. However, I think the Oedipal transition and conflicting loyalties girls experience, particularly in their teenage years, reflects a significant psychological difference between the genders.

Girls, sexual awakening and disturbing thoughts about fathers

When I was a girl of 16 I had a most troubling dream which I think was all about the confusion, conflict and guilt I was experiencing at the time in my own Oedipal triangle.

In the dream I was staying in my grandparents' farmhouse where my family went every year for Christmas. My father and I were alone in the dining room, although I was vaguely aware that the rest of my family were elsewhere in the rambling old house. On the old wooden dining table sat a large cake and beside it lay a gleaming carving knife. My father picked up the knife as if he was planning to cut the cake. I tried to remind him that we always cut the cake when the whole family are present but when he turned to look at me, I found I couldn't speak. As I stared at him and the knife in his hand, his appearance began to transform like a werewolf in a fairy tale; he grew, his figure becoming darker, more menacing, his face becoming strangely contorted. He began advancing towards me with the knife still in his hand and I realised with horror that he was going to rape me.

At that moment I woke up from my dream screaming. My father, who must have heard my screams from the nearby bedroom where he slept with my mother, suddenly burst into my bedroom and switched on the light. He thought a burglar had broken into the house and he had come to rescue me from the attacker. I stared at my father, appalled; the image of him in my nightmare still vivid in my mind. He rather awkwardly asked me if I was alright. I said I was fine, I just had a bad dream. He paused as if not knowing what to do, whether to go back to bed or to offer me comfort. For some reason I noticed the cord dangling from the waist of his dishevelled pyjamas and for a split second I was horrified by the thought that I might accidentally glimpse his penis. The sight of him standing there in his striped pyjamas suddenly disgusted me. I told him again I was fine and asked him to go back to bed. After he had gone I stood a chair in front of my bedroom door. In my confused mind I thought the clatter of the chair would serve as a warning should my father try again to come into my bedroom. The next morning, I awoke to see the chair in front of the door and I felt foolish and ashamed; why would I imagine that my father would come into my bedroom in the middle of the night intent on harming me? Then I remembered my dream.

What could my dream and my fears and fantasies mean? The subject of my nightmare was my fear of my father's incestuous desire. The dream portrayed my father as a Jekyll and Hyde character, the good man I knew and loved was transformed into a bad man I feared. It was as if my father was being consumed by a hidden part of his personality that was dark, malevolent and out of control. I think the dream represented his penis as a knife. But the cake is also important. In the dream I knew it was wrong for my father to cut the cake with only me there; I felt anxious and guilty because the cake should be shared with the family. I think the dream was portraying my fear that my father sexually desired me and my guilt about how this meant I was in some way being disloyal to my mother.

But what had given rise to these fears? I loved my father very much, but he was a complicated and sometimes difficult man. He was secretive, troubled and rarely talked about his feelings. He was given to occasional dark moods when he would withdraw inside of himself, leaving the household shrouded in gloom. I want to be clear: my father never sexually molested me. But I suspect that when I became a teenager he found our relationship as troubling as I did. He appeared to withdraw from me just when I was most insecure about my attractiveness and very much needed him to express his love and approval. The more I sought his approval, particularly his reassurance that I was attractive, the more he withdrew from me. Even on the occasions when he gave me a hug I felt a physical awkwardness between us.

I have no idea what was going on in his sexual imagination, and as he is no longer alive it is impossible to ask him. But as a teenager I was hurt by his apparent loss of interest in me and I couldn't understand what I had done wrong. I think it very likely that my burgeoning sexual awareness disturbed him. I also think it was possible that I sensed his internal struggle with his sexual feelings. My fear, that he may desire me sexually, was a real fear arising from the complicated feelings that seemed to reside in the awkward space between the two of us, feelings that were far too dangerous for either of us to ever speak about.

But why did I dream that he wanted to rape me? Was I afraid that he sexually desired me more than he desired my mother? Or was that my unconscious wish?

In the *Three Essays on the Theory of Sexuality*, Freud writes:

> No doubt the simplest course for the child would be to choose as his sexual objects the same persons whom, since his childhood, he has loved with what may be described as a damped down libido. But by the postponing of sexual maturation, time has been gained in which the child can erect, among other restraints on sexuality, the barrier against incest.
>
> (Freud 1905)

This makes sense to me. I remember, from the age of four, yearning to find ways of making my father happy when he seemed sad or angry and secretly blaming my mother for making him unhappy. These feelings were waves of love; they weren't sexual. But when I hit my teenage years I became awash with strange passions, crushes and sexual desires. The objects of my desire were mainly film stars, pop stars or boys at school. Briefly I was obsessed with our science master. And for a while I even nurtured a passion for the father of one of my school friends and fantasised that he was secretly in love with me. I can see now that he was a sublimation for my father – a safer place for me to project my fantasies, free from the dread of incestuous desire.

Freud said of this adolescent struggle that:

> at the same time as these plain incestuous fantasies are necessarily overcome and repudiated, one of the most significant, but also one of the most painful psychical achievements of the pubertal period [adolescence] is completed: detachment from parental authority.

He is describing a psychosexual rite of passage between puberty and adulthood. This involves a painful but necessary separation from our first love, that is our childhood love and dependence on our opposite sex parent, to enable us to transfer our love, our need to be loved, and our sexual desires to another. This transition is necessary to enable us to achieve our autonomy from our parents and take our place as an adult in the world.

As I said earlier, I don't think it's useful to describe the kind of love and sexual feelings experienced by infants and young children towards their parents as 'incestuous'. In fact, I think it has contributed to a widespread misunderstanding and hostility towards Freud and the Oedipus complex. But when it comes to adolescence, I think my dream is a vivid example of my own unconscious struggle with incestuous sexual desires. I also think the nature of this conflict for girls is even more complex than Freud suggests.

Craving for love and attention and even trying out seduction techniques on her father is normal for a girl in her early teenage years. She needs him to recognise that she is attractive to boost her confidence, which is quite a different thing from wanting him to desire sex with her. I developed from being a tomboy who identified with her father to becoming a pubescent teenage girl practicing my seduction technique on him. Something compelled me to play around in the sexual danger zone between us. But I could do this only so long as at some level I knew that the sexual boundary between us was safely in place.

I cannot rule out the possibility that my dream was fuelled by my rivalry with my mother, and my unconscious desire that my father should find me more sexually desirable than her. My terror and disgust in the dream was my defence against what Freud described as 'plain incestuous fantasies'. But as my dream and my actions on waking demonstrate, there was nothing 'plain' about what I imagined, or fantasised, was going on beneath the surface of my relationship with my father. My dream was telling me that my unconscious was struggling with an awareness of my father, whom I loved, as a sexual being, and my sense of the danger of incestuous desires had not only frightened me but also caused me to feel conflicted and guilty about betraying my mother whom I also loved.

I don't recall feeling much anger or rivalry with my mother as a teenager. My elder sister was the main object of my rivalry, probably because for both me and my sister it was safer to express our anger and destructive feelings towards each other. Our mother was the idealised object at the centre of the family and, because of her frequent depressions, she was too vulnerable to be the object of our rage and rivalry. In my dream, the safety of the family was represented by the cake. It was imperative that the cake was cut fairly into equal portions when the whole family were present to keep the family safe.

But the question remains: Whose incestuous desires was I struggling with? Mine, or my father's? The dream plainly shows that my unconscious was struggling with the troubling possibility that my father, whom I loved and trusted, may have really been fighting to repress his incestuous desires towards me, and subconsciously I was aware of his struggle.

The danger of focussing solely on the internal fantasy world of the child is that it is easy to neglect the very real part the parent may be playing in generating the child's feelings and fantasies. The complexity and the difficulty in all relationships, first with our parents and siblings and later with our partners, lies in sorting out what is our own stuff, what is their stuff, and what is our combined stuff. I was reminded of this when Connie came to see me.

Connie and her flirtatious father

Connie, aged 30, came for therapy because she was isolated and depressed. Apart from going to the university laboratory where she worked as a research scientist, she rarely went out. Also, she was very confused by her relationships with men, so much so that she had decided the only solution was to stop having relationships. She dissolved into tears when she told me this and began frantically apologising. I wondered if her carelessly drab clothes and the way she appeared to be hiding behind her bob of thick black hair were part of her mission to stop men finding her attractive. If so, I guessed it wasn't working. Connie had a childlike innocence about her; it was easy to see why she was attractive to men.

She said she could hardly bring herself to tell me about her problem; she felt so ashamed of the mess she had got herself into. About two years ago she began a relationship with James. He worked with her in the lab. He was a good, kind, loving man and at the time she thought she was in love with him. She also very much wanted a stable relationship. Soon they started living together and she thought she was perfectly happy, until she met James's best friend, Marcus. At first, she disliked Marcus; he was very good-looking, but she thought he was arrogant, selfish and egotistical. She hated the way he treated James like a doormat, but she was also annoyed by the way James idolised him. Soon she began to see James differently; he seemed weak and needy in comparison to Marcus. One day, Marcus came to the flat when James was at the university. Somehow, she ended up in bed with him! She gazed at me with stricken eyes – how could she have done such a thing?

From that day onwards, they continued to have sex secretly without James knowing. The odd thing was that she and Marcus never talked about the fact that they were betraying James. It just didn't seem to be an issue for Marcus. But for Connie the shame was almost unbearable. She realised that she could never tell James about her affair with Marcus; it would break his heart. The only solution she could think of was to end her relationship with James and to stop seeing Marcus. She found herself a place on her own and moved out of the flat she shared with James.

James was broken-hearted, and Connie was consumed by terrible guilt. But still she couldn't stop seeing Marcus, even though she was convinced he only wanted her for sex. For a while she continued to pretend this casual sex thing they had was fine with her when she knew it wasn't fine at all; it was tearing her apart. She couldn't talk to him about things that really mattered to her, like she used to with James. She felt false whenever she was with him, as if she were playing a part; pretending to be the kind of woman she thought he wanted her to be because she was terrified he would lose interest in her. Marcus soon lost interest in her anyway. When she refused to have sex with him, he stopped coming to see her. She said she had even wondered if the sexual thrill for Marcus was precisely the fact that he was having secret sex with his best friend's girlfriend. Sex with her was no longer exciting and forbidden after she left James. Whatever, now she had lost them both. That should have been the end of it. But she still feels as if she's in love with Marcus. She can't stop longing to see him again. Why should a man she didn't even like have this effect on her?

She finished her story and grabbed a handful of tissues to mop up her tears. Her cheeks were burning. She hardly dared to look at me; she was convinced that I was thinking badly of her. I wasn't, I was thinking about her question: what was it about this triangular situation she had got herself into with James and Marcus that had proved so compelling for Connie?

Connie was an only child. She told me she loved her father, although she didn't like him much. He was domineering, arrogant and egotistical. I was struck by how she had used exactly these words to describe Marcus. She said her father despised most people, often calling them stupid and dumb. She particularly hated it when her father called her mother stupid, which he did frequently; it always made Connie uncomfortable. But what troubled Connie most about her father was his obsession with her, particularly his obsession with her body.

She thought his obsession began when she was about ten years old. She remembered a time when her father walked into the bathroom when she was in the bath. Until then, when he had come into the bathroom while she was bathing, she hadn't said anything. But on this day, she knew with absolute certainty that she did mind; she did not want him to see her naked. She asked him to stay out of the bathroom when she was bathing. But he laughed at her and took no notice. It was the same when she asked him to knock before he walked into her bedroom. He simply laughed and refused to understand why she should even want any privacy.

She had loved spending time with him when she was younger. Then it had been as if she and her father were a team; the two of them in league conspiring against her mother who was the outsider. But her feelings changed when she hit puberty. She no longer liked the way he continued to treat her as if she was his little princess and it was just the two of them against her mother. She hated the way he constantly went on about how now 'her tits were growing they bounced under her T-shirt'. And he grabbed her at any opportunity, pinching or slapping her bum as if it was all a huge joke. She was embarrassed by his constant sexual innuendo. She even remembered wondering if he had sexual feelings towards her, but just the thought of such a terrible thing horrified her. At this point in her story she stopped talking and looked appalled and distressed. She said she felt guilty telling me this. She felt as if she were betraying him by telling me. She loved her father and she didn't want me to think badly of him. She was very worried that I might think that he had sexually abused her because he hadn't. It really wasn't like that.

I didn't think that. As I listened to Connie's story, I was reminded of my own adolescent confusion about my father's possible sexual feelings towards me. I was also thinking about how guilty and ashamed Connie felt; it was as if, just by telling me, she had betrayed a terrible secret. But who was it she was afraid of betraying: her father, her mother or both of them?

She said she felt guilty because her father's attention was constantly on her and not on her mother whom he treated like a doormat. This was even though, according to Connie, her mother had always been 'the beautiful one', and Connie was 'the brainy one'. Her father had been determined that she should be brilliant academically and she had usually come top in exams to please him. But at the same time, she had always felt embarrassed about being clever and tried to play it down because she was very afraid of people's envy. She paused for a moment as she thought carefully about her fear of being envied and added: 'I quite like it if men envy me. But I feel awful if it's a woman'.

Now I was wondering about her mother's envy. What can it have been like to be treated like a doormat and ignored by your husband in favour of your beautiful, nubile and extremely clever teenage daughter?

At first Connie insisted that her mother couldn't have been envious of her. Although she was often annoyed with her mother for being weak, not standing up to her father, she knew her mother loved her very much. But then she remembered something about her mother's behaviour that was odd. Unlike Connie's school friends' mothers, her mother never did anything 'girly' with her when she was a teenager; she took no interest in Connie's hair, clothes or make-up. Also, when Connie was about 13 her mother began feeding both her and her father massive amounts of junk food; crisps, chocolate biscuits, cream cakes. Her mother even began over-feeding the cat: 'All three of us, me, my Dad and the cat, became fat and ugly, all except Mum who stayed thin and beautiful. After a couple of years of this I rebelled. I got thin and became a Goth! My parents were appalled when I got a nose ring, and my Dad hated me wearing black all the time.' Connie grinned with delight when she told me this.

It wasn't difficult to see how the conflicting feelings in Connie's Oedipal triangle were still tearing her apart. As a small child, it had been fun and exciting being on her father's 'team' in league against her mother. But when she hit puberty it wasn't fun anymore. Instead the awful fear that he may desire her sexually rose dangerously close to the surface. The mere thought of it both frightened and disgusted her. Also, it came with a gnawing feeling of guilt – even imagining such a terrible thing meant she was betraying her mother. Her father's openly sexualised behaviour towards her, in full view of her mother, exacerbated Connie's guilt and made her still more afraid of her mother's envy. She had described her mother as weak and a bit of a martyr, but her mother's envious attack with food reminded me of the insanely jealous wicked queen in Snow White who tries to get rid of her beautiful daughter by feeding her a poisoned apple.

I suspected that, unconsciously, Connie's feelings towards James and Marcus had been fuelled by these dynamics in her Oedipal triangle. At first, she had been happy with James, a nice man who was secure and reliable and loved her. But when a handsome, dominating and selfish man like her father appeared on the scene, her feelings towards James changed. Now she was sexually attracted to Marcus, she projected onto James the weak, needy and inferior aspects she associated with her mother whom her father treated like a doormat. The entire James-Marcus story was like an action replay of the unconscious psychodynamics in her childhood Oedipal triangle, but with a crucial difference – Marcus was not her father, James was not her mother and the drama was free to unfold to its inevitable climax of sex, betrayal and guilt about the terrible thing she had done.

Whilst in the ancient tragedy, when Oedipussy was confronted by the shock of what she had done she gouged out her eyes, Connie's self-punishment had been her self-imposed exile in a lonely life without men or sexual relationships. Telling her story in therapy helped her to make sense of her story which alleviated her guilt and freed her from her punishing isolation. After some time, she was able to face the world again and resume her search for the kind of loving relationship she wanted.

A few years later I emailed her to ask for her permission to use her story for this book. I attached this piece to the email. A few days later her reply pinged into my inbox. She said she now had 'a wonderful and very supportive boyfriend.' She had even shared with him the piece I had written about our work together in therapy: 'It served a useful purpose in helping us to understand each other a little better. I think if I had met him before we did the work together I would have run away from him because he was "too nice"'.

Fantasies or memories of abuse? An important distinction

It's not difficult to understand why Connie was so anxious about telling me about her father's sexualised behaviour towards her. Admitting to dreams or fantasies that include sexual feelings about our parents, or even fears about sexual feelings our parents may have about us, is almost impossible without arousing powerful and deeply disturbing fears about incest.

Incest is a universal taboo for obvious reasons to do with the species' need to maintain a healthy gene pool, and the lasting psychological trauma inflicted on children by parents, older siblings or close relatives who sexually abuse them. Nevertheless, research has revealed that incest is shockingly common in societies worldwide. There are no statistics regarding what goes on in the imaginations of adults who do not act on their fantasies or temptations. But I think we can assume that rather more adults than we like to think may have secretly struggled with sexual feelings they have not acted on towards their own children or towards young people in their care.

Many of Freud's female patients who came to him suffering from what was then labelled as 'hysteria' (nowadays the diagnosis would be post-traumatic stress disorder, psychotic episodes, or personality disorder) told him about the sexual abuse they had endured in childhood. Their abuser was most often their father, a close relative or someone in their family circle. Male patients also had severe psychological symptoms rooted in memories of sexual abuse by their mothers, caregivers, or parent substitutes such as teachers or priests. It wasn't only Freud's patients who had suffered sexual abuse in childhood. His colleague, the psychoanalyst Carl Jung, confided in a letter to Freud that 'as a boy I was a victim of a sexual assault by a man I once worshipped,' that had left him with an 'an abominable feeling' (1907). Ferenczi, another close colleague, traced his own psychological wounds back to the emotional and sexual traumas inflicted chiefly by his mother and his nursemaid which Ferenczi believed had resulted in his compulsion to masturbate four or five times a day (Rudnytsky 2002).

The problem for Freud was that when initially he spoke publicly about the numbers of his clients suffering from severe psychological symptoms resulting from childhood sexual abuse, he was attacked. This is not so surprising, as he had plunged headlong into taboo territory in the highly conservative climate of late 19th-century Vienna. Consequently, he appeared to change his mind and began to interpret his clients' accounts as 'fantasies' and unresolved sexual longings. In contrast, Ferenczi never wavered in his belief that his clients were telling the truth, probably because he was a survivor of sexual abuse himself and he knew too well the profound impact it had had on his own mental health. But this stand may well have contributed to his life-long marginalisation in the psychoanalytic community (Bodenheimer 2010). Rows about this contentious issue and what Freud did or did not believe have continued in the psychoanalytic community ever since. The tragic repercussions for victims of sexual abuse in childhood have been great. Subsequent generations of Freud's followers were taught in their psychoanalytic institutes that memories of incestuous abuse were likely to be unconscious repressed Oedipal wishes, with the result that their clients suffered the additional trauma of not being believed by their psychoanalysts.

Over the years, so-called false memory syndrome has routinely been used in court by lawyers to discredit victims of sexual abuse. Psychotherapists, who believed their clients' accounts, have been accused of 'planting fantasies' in their clients' minds. Abusers always look for a way out, and what better defence than to point the finger of blame at either their accuser, by asserting that they must have been fantasising, or their psychotherapist who must have caused them to tell their 'disgusting lies'. It's easier to accuse victims of being 'hysterical' or mad than to believe their shocking stories.

Most psychotherapists I know see clients who have been sexually abused. Often the perpetrators are fathers, mothers, step-parents, siblings or close relatives, or they were abused by parent figures such as boarding school teachers or priests. We need only to do the maths and extrapolate from my relatively small circle of colleagues to realise that the sexual abuse of children continues to be one of the most common causes of serious mental illness in adults.

But where does this leave the important distinction between memories of incestuous sexual abuse and memories of sexual feelings, fantasies or dreams featuring a parent that are a normal part of the Oedipal stage of children and young people's psychosexual development? Nowhere really. If anything, the pendulum has swung in the other direction. It is still almost impossible to talk about sexual fears, fantasies or dreams involving parents, such as those experienced by Connie, or my own dream of my father, without the fear of being misunderstood. Whereas, as we have seen, such fantasies and fears are a natural and important part of some young people's psychosexual development representing their struggle to separate from their childhood love for their father or mother to be free to love another.

4 Love and attachment and why they matter

Falling in love, settling into the more complex business of loving and being loved, or surviving rejection and facing the daunting prospect of starting over if the relationship isn't working is for many of us an emotional roller coaster. But why is it that for some people the whole terrain of finding a partner and forming intimate loving relationships is experienced as an emotional danger zone requiring all sorts of defence or attack strategies, including resisting intimacy entirely? I think John Bowlby, a child and family psychiatrist and psychoanalyst, provided some important answers.

The origins of attachment theory

Bowlby, the originator of attachment theory, devoted his life to understanding the emotional roots of our ability, or inability, to give love and be loved, and all the emotions that are aroused by what he called our attachment system. He firmly believed that along with food and sex, equally important for survival are a secure base and our ability to form attachments with others. Like Freud, he was convinced that the key to what makes us who we are lies in our early childhood development. But rather than rely on the dreams, fantasies and childhood memories of his patients, Bowlby was interested in looking at the effect on children of the actual behaviour of parents and care-givers towards them. He was particularly concerned by the effect on the children of abuse, neglect, separation and loss:

> Such experiences greatly increase a child's fear of losing his mother, increase his demands for her presence and also his anger at her absences, and may also lead him to despair of ever having a secure and loving relationship with anyone.
>
> (Bowlby 1988)

I think his own early life tells us a lot about why he was so drawn to this area of research.

Bowlby was born early in the 20th century, a time when it was typical in upper-middle-class English families, like the Bowlbys, for children to see their mothers only for a brief time each day; if they were lucky, for an hour after tea. Consequently, young Bowlby became very attached to his nursemaid, Minnie, who had looked after him since he was born. When he was four years old, his beloved Minnie suddenly left the family. Maybe she found more lucrative employment or got married. Whatever, the effect on Bowlby was profound. He later said that for him, losing Minnie was the equivalent of the tragic loss of a mother. This wasn't his only painful separation. Some years later he was sent away to a boys' boarding school. In *Separation: Anxiety and Anger* (1973), he says this was a terrible time for him. He is also reputed to have said he wouldn't send a dog away to boarding school aged seven.

What are the basic concepts of attachment theory? For the first few years of our life, our secure base is largely dependent on the nature of our attachment to our mother or primary care-giver, in Bowlby's case this was Minnie, his nanny. If our mother is responsive to our needs, we feel safe enough and courageous enough to explore the world around us and to form attachments with others, knowing she will be there for us when we return from our adventures. The securely attached child is therefore likely to develop what Bowlby called a positive internal working model, which means they feel good about themselves, they have a sense of emotional well-being, and a solid foundation for forming intimate, satisfying relationships with others throughout life. Problems arise if our mother or care-giver is cold, neglectful, insensitive, inconsistent, unreliable, cruel, abusive or abandoning like Minnie who, from the point of view of a four-year-old child, suddenly disappeared one day as if she had died.

If a child's sense of being loved, protected and secure is frequently or constantly under threat, they resort to primitive defensive strategies in a struggle to manage their confusing, painful and frightening emotions. If these primitive defensive strategies become entrenched, the child forms a negative internal working model of its self and of others, which can have a life-long impact on the ability to form fulfilling, loving relationships.

> The child, and later the adult, becomes afraid to allow himself to become attached to anyone for fear of a further rejection with all the agony, the anxiety, and the anger to which that would lead. As a result, there is a massive block against his expressing or even feeling his natural desire for a close trusting relationship, for care, comfort, and love.
>
> (Bowlby 1988)

In the 1970s Mary Ainsworth, a student of Bowlby's, devised an experiment known as the Strange Situation, which provided additional evidence to support attachment theory. The Strange Situation was beautifully simple. The idea was to observe the behaviour of infants when their mothers or primary care-givers left them alone in a room with a stranger and to observe the infants' behaviour when their mothers returned. From the experiment Ainsworth concluded that there were three attachment styles: secure, insecure-ambivalent, and insecure-avoidant. What fascinates me is how easy it is to recognise in Ainsworth's observations of the children similar patterns of behaviour in some adult relationships.

Luckily most of the infants Ainsworth studied were securely attached. They played and explored freely whilst their mother was in the room, using her as a secure base. They were upset when their mother left and avoided contact with the stranger. But when their mother returned, they were happy to see her and quickly regained their sense of well-being. Ainsworth concluded that these infants were confident that their attachment figure was responsive to their needs and would be there for them if they were distressed.

Infants whose attachment style was insecure-ambivalent tended to be clingy and difficult to comfort even before their mothers left the room. They avoided the stranger and appeared fearful of her. When mother returned, they either appeared helpless or angrily pushed her away. These infants were both more dependent and more rejecting of their mothers. Ainsworth thought this was a response to the mother's ambivalent behaviour towards her child. If the mother's behaviour was inconsistent, erratic and unpredictable, her child became so preoccupied with her that it lacked the necessary sense of security to explore its surroundings.

In contrast, the infants whose attachment style was insecure-avoidant didn't appear to depend on their mother as a secure base when they explored their new surroundings in the room, they didn't seem to be upset when their mother left them alone with the stranger and they showed little interest when their mother returned. They appeared to be very independent of their mother physically and emotionally. But Ainsworth realised that these children had learnt to be self-sufficient because their mother was rarely there for them when they needed her, and if she was there, she was more likely to ignore or reject their needs.

A fourth category, insecure-disorganised, was added later. The children displayed a bewildering mixture of ambivalent and avoidant behaviours indicating that they were extremely insecure and deeply troubled by their relationship to their mother or care-giver.

Attachment theory and sexual relationships

It's easier to observe the behaviour of mothers and infants in laboratory conditions than it is to carry out scientific research on the feelings and behaviour of adults in the privacy of their intimate love relationships. However, since the 1980s, researchers have been looking at the impact attachment styles developed in childhood may have on adult love relationships.

Chris Fraley and Phillip Shaver described two common, easily recognisable and distinctly different defensive strategies employed by people with insecure attachment styles, and negative working models of themselves and others, in managing their emotions in intimate relationships. The first, which is like an insecure infant's anxious-ambivalent attachment style, is when the defensive strategies are hyperactive. Their emotional system is constantly on the alert due to an imagined or paranoid threat of betrayal, abandonment, or simply not being loved as they think they should be. Their behaviour is variously clinging, controlling and/or actively coercive, to get their partner to be responsive, to pay attention and to provide better care. The problem for these people, and their partners, is that rather than achieving the aim of making the relationship more secure this strategy exacerbates the conflict in the relationship, heightens the distress and reinforces their sense of insecurity.

The second is like an insecure infant's avoidant attachment style. The defensive strategies employed involve inhibiting or dampening down emotions to maintain a physical or emotional distance from others, and to avoid intimacy and the danger of dependency at all costs. Bowlby originally called this defensive strategy 'compulsive self-reliance'.

Fraley and Shaver hypothesised that people with hyperactive anxious-ambivalent defensive strategies are more likely to use sex as a way of gaining the acceptance, love and security they desire. But due to their anxiety and insecurity they find it more difficult to enjoy sex. Whereas people with avoidant defensive strategies are more likely to block intimacy by remaining emotionally distant, engage only in short-term sexual encounters, or prefer the self-reliance of masturbation. A 2002 study found that avoidant people engaged less frequently in sex with partners, and they reported masturbating more frequently. Fraley and Shaver note how this solitary activity fits well with Bowlby's concept of 'compulsive self-reliance'. Masturbation can be a way of avoiding anxieties about intimacy and vulnerability. Another way of avoiding anxieties about the vulnerability of intimacy is to use sex as a way of gaining control over their partner and to bolster their self-esteem. Rather than empathising with their partner's feelings, they keep the focus on their own narcissistic needs.

Fraley and Shaver also cite studies which reveal some interesting gender differences. Men who have an insecure anxious-avoidant style tend to have less frequent sexual activity with partners. Whereas women who have an insecure anxious-avoidant style tend to start sexual activity at a younger age than normal and have increased sexual activity generally. Of course, this could also be a sign that insecure girls and women have such a low self-esteem they use sex as a way of feeling good about themselves, at least temporarily, by reassuring themselves that they are desirable to men.

All of this might suggest that people who have a secure attachment style and positive 'working models' of themselves and others are more likely to be comfortable with intimacy, self-disclosure and interdependence. In other words, securely attached adults are more likely to enjoy satisfying sexual lives. However, we all have survival strategies and defences which kick in, consciously or unconsciously, in our intimate relationships. We will also have formed a positive, or negative, internal working model, often as a response to our childhood family relationships. But our attachment style, whatever it is, will necessarily respond and react to our partner's attachment style. For instance, if we have a secure attachment system but find ourselves with a partner who is ambivalent or avoidant, our responses may begin to resemble their avoidant model as a way of defending ourselves. We might assume that securely attached people will choose securely attached partners, but in the world of love and sexual relationships, matters of sexual desire and who we choose as a partner, are rarely that straightforward. It could be that the adventurous spirit and curiosity of the securely attached person leads them to take greater risks with their choice of sexual partners, only to find themselves deeply attached to a partner who is cold and distant or ambivalent and even abusive. Their ability to trust others and their sense of loyalty born of their early secure attachments may make it even harder for them to break free from an unhappy relationship.

As a psychotherapist, I am very aware that my relationship with a client is also an attachment relationship. If the therapy is going well, all the attachment dynamics described by Bowlby are alive, and sometimes kicking, in the here and now in the consulting room. As the therapist, I am my client's secure base and the consulting room is, or should be, experienced as their safe place where they can explore difficult, unhappy and painful aspects of their past and present life with me as care-giver, providing empathy, support and understanding, and challenging them when necessary, however hard that is. I frequently find myself thinking about a client's positive or negative internal working models of themselves and others, including me, and their defensive systems and attachment styles, particularly if they seem to be oscillating, as they sometimes do, between anxious dependency and angry self-reliance, and all the positions in between. And, like all care-givers, therapists sometimes get things wrong, or are not there when needed, or go on holiday just when the client has a crisis.

But I also have reservations about attachment theory. I worry that it can cause struggling mothers to feel like guilty failures. They look up attachment styles on the Internet and become convinced that they are ruining their child's life. They are desperately torn between attending to their own very real and pressing needs and the attachment needs of their child. Will they damage their child if they send their child to nursery because they need to go back to work; they are missing their career, or they have pressing financial needs, or they are a single parent and can hardly cope, or they are depressed, or bored stuck at home with children all day? Attachment theory feeds into their guilt, they think they ought to be a perfect mother, and instead they are struggling to be good enough, which is all any of us can be in the difficult business of real life. The emphasis in attachment theory on mothers and care-givers, mostly female, seems to give dads a free pass. Some dads say they want to share equally in the childcare, but work structures prevent them from doing so. But even dads who provide the income whilst mums stay at home with the children have a shared responsibility for whether the children feel secure or experience the family as a cold, unloving or dangerous place.

Family life is complicated. Stuff happens that changes us. Families may split up, loved ones may die, we may be bullied or abused at school or in our social network. Life's vicissitudes continue to affect us deeply throughout childhood, adolescence and adulthood. Human resilience and sensitivity vary from person to person. We may have been badly hurt in infancy or childhood, but reparative relationships may be formed with a grandparent, a teacher, a caring friend, even a psychotherapist or counsellor, which has the capacity to revive our ability to love and trust others. To add to the complexity, our culture and environment will also have a profound effect on our intimate relationships and our sexual lives.

I have an aversion to fitting people into four neat pigeonholes. It might satisfy a craving for simple explanations to conclude that if human beings can be categorised into four attachment styles developed in infancy, we have the key to understanding what's going wrong in our intimate sexual relationships. However, even some leading proponents of attachment theory have begun to look again at the Oedipal triangle and accept that the subject of adult love and sexual relationships is far too complex for a single theory.

Kieran's terror of being abandoned

The fear of being abandoned is so great for some people that it blights all their intimate relationships. As soon as a new relationship begins, they become beset by anxieties about how the other person sees them and whether they can trust this person not to leave them. Their strategies for defending themselves against what feels like an inevitability can become increasingly convoluted. The defences they devise to save themselves from being hurt and abandoned eat away at whatever is good in the relationship and eventually cause the very thing they most dread. This reinforces the firmly held belief that there must be something so bad about them that all their relationships will be doomed to failure. This was Kieran's story.

My first thought when Kieran, in his mid-thirties, greeted me with a warm, polite smile, was how good-looking he was. He was tall and slim with dark hair, sparkling blue eyes and stylishly dressed. It was easy to see why, with his relaxed charm, he was an experienced manager in an expensive London hotel. But Kieran didn't see himself like this at all. He was convinced there was something wrong with his looks, and he had always believed there was something bad about him.

Soon after he arrived for his first session, he became flustered and began to cry. He said he was very embarrassed, he hardly ever cried, and he didn't know why he was crying now. I asked him what he had been thinking about when he started to cry. He said his first thought when he sat down was that he felt like a small child with me. He then remembered being sent to primary school when he was five. He said he had been a very bad child, disruptive and completely out of control. At the school there was a woman teacher whom he liked very much, but whenever she tried to put her arm around him to comfort him and give him some affection, he pushed her away. That was what he had thought of when he sat down and looked at me; he remembered pushing her away when all he had really wanted was for her to love him. He still feels guilty about it. But he couldn't understand why he remembered it now; it didn't make any sense.

I suggested that maybe he wanted to push me away, like he had pushed away his teacher, when all he really wanted was for me to care for him? He nodded and blew his nose loudly. He said whenever he started a relationship, he always found himself wanting to push his new boyfriend away. But this wasn't a relationship, it was therapy and it would be silly to try and push me away when he really needed to me to help him.

Kieran's parents split up when he was 18 months old. He had no memory of his mother leaving him with his father, but as a child he believed that it was his fault they divorced because he had cried so much as a baby. The agreement was they would each take one of the children: 'They assumed a boy would be happier with his Dad and a girl with her Mum – forgetting that I was only eighteen months old and still needed my Mum! But my battered, weak Mum just agreed with whatever my Dad wanted,' Kieran said.

It sounded to me as if his battered mother would have agreed to anything to get away from his bullying father. But whatever the reason, his mother left him behind. The inevitable outcome was that little Kieran, now abandoned by his mother, spent the next few months crying even more. His mother told him much later that when she came to visit him, he used to sit in the hall hugging her shoes to prevent her from leaving again. Even Kieran's father, whom Kieran described as a cold, unfeeling man, who probably had no idea what to do with a baby, had to admit that the arrangement wasn't working. Their solution was to swap the children again; this time Kieran's five-year-old sister was left with Dad and Kieran's mother took him home with her.

Kieran's earliest childhood memory was when he was two years old. His mother was tucking him up in the cot in the corner of her room in his grandparents' house. He remembered feeling happy at last because he was with his mother. But his happiness didn't last. His mother was young and desperate for the life she had missed out on when she was married to his father. For the next five years Kieran's life with his deeply troubled mother was chaotic and frightening. She joined a hippy cult and took her young son to live with her in various communal apartments where she had a room. 'She drank, she took lots of drugs, and even slept with knives under the bed, so I have no idea how she took care of me. Every so often, she would dump me with my grandma and disappear.'

'Knives under the bed?' I asked.

'I guess she thought there were some dangerous people in that house. I don't really remember. I remember feeling safer with my grandmother.'

Kieran's much-loved grandmother at least provided him with some stability, whilst his mother's erratic lifestyle and frequent disappearances were traumatic. No wonder Kieran wanted to push me away like he had pushed away his primary school teacher and his boyfriends. This was his defence against his all-consuming fear of being abandoned again. He very much wanted psychotherapy to help him with his dark depressions, but the conflict he felt was acute. What if he allowed himself to get attached to me and I abandoned him one day like his mother had? That would be too much for him to bear.

This fear was present for much of Kieran's therapy. He would arrive for his sessions and tell me he was worried about disappointing me. Or I must be thinking he's wasting my time and getting bored with him. Or I would find a better job and pass him on to another therapist. He was plagued by similar thoughts about his boyfriend, Oliver, who he was convinced was going to dump him. He had always been afraid his boyfriends were going to get fed up with him and leave him for another man.

'Like you think I am going to get fed up with you?' I asked.

'Yes.'

'Like your mother left you when you were little?'

'Yes.'

'Because you cried?'

'Yes.'

'It is normal for babies to cry, just like it is normal for clients to cry sometimes in therapy.'

'Maybe,' he admitted reluctantly, 'but I still don't like the feeling of losing control. And I don't want to be angry with my mother any more. Although sometimes I really hate her.' This time the tears gushed out of his eyes. He grabbed tissues and shook as he tried to control them. 'I feel so guilty,' he mumbled, 'I can't believe I said that. How terrible, to say you hate your mother.'

'Just because we love someone doesn't mean we can't hate them sometimes,' I suggested.

'I know, but sometimes I think my mother is a really bad person. She gets so angry her face changes. She says hurtful things like how me and my sister have ruined her life. Last time I went home to stay with her, when I was so depressed, I couldn't get out of bed. For two beautiful weeks she was marvellous, strong, caring and then she suddenly became very angry with me and said she would have been better off if she'd never had children.'

He fell silent and stared out of the window at a plane passing overhead. I found myself wondering if he was wishing he was up there high above the clouds escaping from all the terrible things in world below.

Kieran was obsessed with the thought that he was unlovable because he was 'wicked'. One day I tried to tackle his conviction head on.

'Kieran, I don't know what you mean by "being wicked". . . . I'm thinking of the time you told me about when you were a small boy in primary school. What was that small boy feeling?'

'That's easy,' he said, 'he was very, very angry.'

'Why was he angry?'

'Because he was hurt. He wanted to be loved but pushed people away because he didn't believe anyone could love him because he was bad. He was bad; his behaviour was so awful no one could get near him.'

'I don't think he was bad. I think he was a very distressed child who was angry because he had been abandoned by his mother when he couldn't possibly have done anything bad to deserve being abandoned. The question for us is: can he begin to love that child and stop giving him such a tough time?'

Kieran's face suddenly broke into a broad grin: 'That is just about the worst cliché you have ever come up with.'

We both laughed. Kieran suddenly looked thoughtful. He had just remembered, he said, two times when he was happy with his mother when he was a kid. Once he and his mother were walking through a park laughing together. His mother was holding his hand and they were dancing about kicking up the autumn leaves. And another time they were just having fun stealing apples from a farmer's orchard.

As he left the session he turned and gave me a little wave.

The session felt like a turning point and, naively, I began to think we were making progress. I was right in a way: that session did mark a change. But not the change I had hoped for. I felt the change as soon as he arrived for his next session. He had a whole new defensive strategy in place. He grinned at me as soon as he came in the room and announced that he was feeling very good today: 'I split up with Oliver. That feels good because I'm not worried any more about Oliver leaving me.' He stopped speaking and looked at me bashfully. 'But now we are together again because Oliver cried and said he was desperate to have me back.'

'So, splitting up and then getting back together changed things?'

'Yes,' Kieran said firmly. 'Now I'm in control. I'm still worried about the jealousy and the competition with Oliver. I hate the way he always gets the attention when we go out together because he is so good looking. But I have a plan. Oliver and I are going to Spain together for a sexy holiday.'

He stopped speaking, looked at me and frowned.

'What plan?' I prompted him.

He smiled. 'I'm not sure I should tell you. I don't want to shock you.'

'It's quite hard to shock a psychotherapist.'

'Okay. The plan is to find someone for threesome sex.'

'And Oliver's test?'

'I will find out if Oliver acts like we are a proper couple. Or if he competes with me for attention. Oliver mustn't flirt with anyone and mustn't be disloyal. These are the two most important things.'

'Does Oliver know he is being tested?'

He smiled. 'If Oliver knew it wouldn't be a proper test. I can't stand it when Oliver is disloyal. For instance, if Oliver argues with me in public, I get very angry. I hate it if anyone, even a stranger, sees that bad things are going on in private. Like when I was a kid living with my mother, I didn't want anyone to know what was really going on. It was very important that everything was perfect on the outside.'

I noticed that again he had again slipped seamlessly from talking about Oliver to talking about his relationship with his mother. I asked him to tell me more about what had gone on at home with his mother. Did she have boyfriends? Were they getting the attention that Kieran wanted?

'Yes,' Kieran said reluctantly. 'That question feels like a knife in my stomach. I'm ashamed and disgusted when I think about it. I don't want to talk about it because it makes me feel bad. But I suppose, as this is therapy, I should. Yes, she had boyfriends, lots of boyfriends. She used to bring them home to the room we lived in. It only had one bed. I had to share it with my Mum. She had sex with them in that bed. She thought I was asleep, but I wasn't. I was very scared. I thought these men were hurting her. She was very noisy, and I didn't understand it at all. Even then, I was about the age of five or six, I think I knew I was gay. I used to open my eyes and peep at the man's naked body. That's what I was interested in, not my Mum's body. Her naked body disgusted me. Another disgusting thing my Mum used to do was call me "brat" all the time like it was my name. I hated that. But when I was thirteen, I told her to stop. "Stop calling me brat, how would you like it if I called you pussy?" She laughed and lifted her skirt and showed me everything. It was disgusting. I can't stand thinking about it, even now. She used to touch me, stroke my arms and talk about how I was becoming a man. I hated her touching me like that. I still don't like it when she touches me.'

'It sounds like she was flirting with you?'

He didn't want to think about his mother flirting with him. But talking about his mother's boyfriends had touched a nerve and he didn't want to stop. He went on to tell me about the time when he was four years old. She took him with her on holiday to Greece. His mother flirted with the Greek waiters. He smiled. 'It's so tacky, being on holiday and flirting with the waiters. It's just the kind of thing I would do on holiday. Anyway, she got off with a waiter and he came with us to the beach the next day. We were sitting on the beach and Mum and the waiter went for a swim. They swam away and disappeared out of sight. I was left alone on the beach screaming. I panicked. I thought they were never coming back. On the day we were leaving for the airport that guy put me on the back of his motorbike and took me for a ride. I screamed and screamed. I was terrified. I thought I would never see my Mum again, she was going to fly home without me.'

'You thought she had abandoned you again.'

We sat in silence for a while. 'Yes,' he said finally, 'but she was only trying to have a good time while she was still young. It must have been hard for her with a little kid trailing along. I don't want to hate her for it.'

'Kieran, the point of therapy is not to encourage you to hate your mother. But we are trying to understand your relationship with your mother and how it is now affecting your relationship with Oliver. I am thinking that maybe you are still trying to protect yourself from the hurt and betrayal you felt when you were a boy and your mother went off with her boyfriends. Maybe you are afraid that Oliver might behave like your mother when you are in Spain together? But instead of talking to Oliver about your fears you are secretly setting a kind of honey trap for Oliver. The trap is the test and it is a test that you know Oliver will probably fail and then you will feel hurt, like you were hurt when your mother went off with the waiter. But at the same time as being hurt you will also feel triumphant, vindicated. Better to have proved that Oliver doesn't really love you than to be in the more unbearable place where you are eaten up by suspicion and mistrust because you can't believe that Oliver loves you however much he says he does.'

I paused and looked at Kieran.'Of course, there is an alternative.'

'What's that?' he asked, doubtfully.

'Dump the test and try talking to Oliver about what you are afraid of.'

He grinned. I had the feeling he wasn't ready for the alternative.

Kieran appeared to have switched from his previous hyperactive, ambivalent attachment style, when he was consumed by a constant, unbearable anxiety about Oliver abandoning or betraying him, to an avoidant attachment style which involved dampening down his emotions to gain distance and enable him to take control. He liked this new feeling of being in control and he wasn't going to give it up that easily.

A few weeks later he arrived for his session, smiled triumphantly and announced that he had been very bad; he had betrayed Oliver. He had a secret rendezvous with another man. He had also left his mobile phone where Oliver could see a text from his new lover. Oliver was very upset when he found out. Kieran insisted that what was so bad about his behaviour was that it was deliberate – he was enjoying hurting Oliver! And he was feeling happy! Now could I understand what he meant when he said he was a wicked person?

To give me further proof of how bad he was he said he had decided to withdraw from sex with Oliver. When they were apart, they talked all the time on the phone; they continued to spend most of their free time together; they slept together in the same bed most nights, but Kieran refused to have sex with Oliver because if they had sex it would mean they had a future together. I asked why they didn't have a future together anyway if they loved each other, particularly as Kieran had said that he wanted a long-term, loving relationship more than anything? It sounded to me as if he was trying to sabotage the relationship. Kieran could see this. But he didn't want to separate from Oliver and he didn't want to go back to how it was when he was depressed and jealous and frightened all the time that Oliver would leave him. At least now he felt in control of the relationship even if being in control meant he was being hurtful and bad.

Kieran was either the vulnerable, out of control, victim, terrified of being abandoned by the person he loved. Or he was 'being bad' by taking control and doing the very things he was most afraid of being done to him; hurting and betraying the person he loved. I think the pleasure he said he felt when hurting Oliver was his way of finding relief from his anxiety that Oliver would hurt him – so long as he was the one inflicting hurt, he felt safer but that also reinforced his insistence that he was a 'wicked person'.

Compared to all the wickedness out there in the world, I didn't think Kieran's misdemeanours rated very high on the badness scale. But Kieran was obstinately determined to hold onto his belief that he was a bad person whatever reassurance I gave him to the contrary.

I think Kieran was in the grips of what Ronald Fairbairn called 'the moral defence'. Fairbairn was a Scottish psychoanalyst who worked in the 1930s with children who had been taken into care to protect them from neglectful and abusive parents. His ideas were later to influence Bowlby and attachment theory. When Fairbairn talked to the children in care, he was puzzled by their insistence that it was their own fault, not their parents' fault, that they had been neglected and abused. Deep down they believed that they had been treated badly because they were bad. Fairbairn realised that children have a great need to hold onto an idealised image of their parents as essentially good. This need was so great they had convinced themselves that they deserved their parents' bad behaviour. He called this defence mechanism 'the moral defence'. If the children believed that they themselves were bad, they could maintain the fantasy of their parents as good people who really loved them despite everything that had been done to them. This fantasy good parent was essential for the children's sense of security and, most of all, their hope for the future. Without it all they would have left would be the awful hopelessness of feeling abandoned and unloved in a cruel world.

The task Kieran and I faced together throughout his therapy was to convince him to let go of this defensive system. Or to put it another way, to enable him to experience through our relationship in the consulting room that he was safe enough to let go of this bad-child part of himself and believe that there was hope, he was lovable and good enough to stop sabotaging all his love relationships including his relationship with me.

This is an email Kieran sent to me many years after his therapy ended. In the email he told me about the voluntary work he had done for the National Autistic Society with an 11-year-old boy called Henry. He told me that Henry was like how he had been as a child. He said: 'I was very closed up and reclusive as a child. I didn't fit in. Working with Henry I saw a side of myself that I had never seen before – a calm and protective side. Dealing with someone who has Asperger Syndrome can be very hard and he was very good at trying to manipulate me to get what he wanted, but he didn't, and I think he felt good that he knew I was strong and had boundaries.'

His email made me smile; Kieran could have been talking about the work we did together in therapy, only this time Kieran was the therapist and Henry was Kieran as a child. At the end of the email he said: 'It was a hard therapy and I was sometimes intimidated by you – in a good way. I needed to feel that way. I'm still not perfect and that's okay and I still have some self-esteem issues, but I can live with that. But I'm not "bad", and you were the one who taught me that.'

Adele, the bad email and the lump of coal

Adele usually appeared bright, colourful and cheerful when she arrived for her sessions, but as I soon learnt, this was her work persona. She was in her mid-forties and ran her own busy yoga studio; I'm sure her clients would never have guessed what was going on in her private world behind the scenes.

She came to see me because, as she put it, she 'needed to know how to turn feelings of romantic love into friendship love'. The problem was, she was in love with her best friend and she was afraid of losing him. 'I know you don't have the answer,' she added, quickly, 'although it would be great if you had a pill to fix it.' Her burst of laughter was infectious.

Adele had been in love with her best friend, Vince, for the past six years and she had been telling me about it in therapy for over a year, ever since she had sent Vince an email; the 'Bad Email' she called it. She said she had sent it in 'a crazy hissy-fit. Late at night I had suddenly found myself writing down all my real feelings for him in this email and then I just pressed send!'

These were not sentimental feelings of love and adoration, these were her conflicted feelings of love, desire, hate, fury and jealousy of the attention Vince was constantly giving to other women. Her email revealed the secret that she had kept from him for the past six years – that although he thought she was his best friend and she played the role to perfection, in fact she was secretly in love with him. This secret love was driving her crazy. She said it was like a horrible addiction. She needed to give him up, but how could she if he kept contacting her, like any friend would, wanting to call in for a coffee at the drop of a hat, or asking her to go out for a drink with him to talk about his work, his health, his love life or whatever they always talked about in their friendship?

It seemed to me that this friendship was somewhat one-sided. Adele listened to Vince, she reassured him endlessly if he was miserable, she contributed ideas and made suggestions for whatever subject he wanted to talk about, she laughed at his jokes and sometimes made jokes of her own. She was his happy-go-lucky friend, always there for him when he felt like talking. But the hidden truth was that the intense anxiety of longing for him to get in touch only left her when they were in some form of communication – telephone, text, emails, whatever – for Adele any form of communication was better than the emptiness of wishing she was with him. Each time he got in touch, something she needed was satisfied just enough to quell her desperation. The crumbs of affection he gave her were just enough to calm the cravings of this starving woman.

But late one night something happened; she turned into a 'crazy lady and wrote him that horrible, furious desperate email.' Her passion, her despair, her craving, her jealousy, her love poured forth in a jumble of words with a terrible intensity. That was how she described it to me, 'the horrible email, the bunny-boiler email'.

'Adele, I've read the email,' I reminded her – she had brought me a printout of the email to read. It was true, it was a confused jumble of her real feelings, passionate and loving and desperate and angry and sad. But it was not a 'bunny-boiler email'. It was not mad. It was not an email from a crazy woman threatening to do him harm. That was just her way of hating herself for writing it, because the act of writing it meant she had revealed her true self to him. This was what she was finding so unbearable. The question was, why was she so ashamed of her true feelings of love? Why should these feelings be shameful and kept hidden?

She knew the answer immediately, 'Because I might lose him. Better to have him as a friend than not at all.'

I reminded her that she sent him the email some time ago and far from running away from her, he was behaving the same as he always had. She had given me a blow-by-blow account over the months. He had received her email, and he had told her he was angry about it and he didn't want her to send him emails like that ever again. And then their friendship had continued as if nothing had happened. He called her up or came to see her when he felt like a chat; he told her about the other women he fancied; he cancelled dinner they had planned together, even if she had spent the whole day cooking, because something, or somebody, more interesting had turned up; he texted her from his holidays abroad telling her what a great time he was having without so much as asking how she was. She was still in the same position in relation to him, only it was worse now she had the 'Bad Email' to add to her catalogue of shame. One more thing to beat herself up about. What she was refusing to see was how her shame was blinding her to Vince's narcissism.

She frowned, she didn't like my suggestion that Vince might be narcissistic. She suddenly became a protective mother hen. She told me I didn't understand him; he was kind to her sometimes, he did little things for her around the house like fix her computer or put up shelves. And he'd had a tough childhood, his father walked out when he was little, and he had a difficult relationship with his mother, which made her wonder if this was why he found intimacy hard.

Adele was never happier than when she was talking about Vince and she would happily have spent all her sessions psychoanalysing him. But I was determined to keep the focus on her. 'Adele, I am sorry that I suggested Vince was narcissistic, I have never met him, and I only have what you tell me to go on. But if you received an email from a friend, like the one you sent Vince, how would you have responded?'

She reluctantly conceded that she would have felt very concerned about the pain her friend was in and wanted to help in some way, even if that meant ending their friendship for a while. The hard thing for Adele to accept was that she had confessed her real feelings to Vince and he'd had so little empathy or regard for her feelings that, rather than be concerned for her, he had been angry with her and demanded that she never send him an email like that again. He had ignored her feelings entirely and tucked her back into the friendship box where he wanted her to stay.

Adele was crying now. This was hard for her to hear. My heart went out to her. I felt her vulnerability and her need to be loved. In that moment, I felt love for her. 'Adele,' I asked, as gently as I could, 'can you tell me about the feelings behind your tears?'

She looked at me sadly. 'It's about the shame. You saying I don't have to be ashamed of that email, I don't have to be ashamed of my feelings. It's alright to have those feelings. I suppose it's hearing you say that I am not bad. That made me cry.'

Something real was now happening in the room between us. It was about my recognition of her true feelings and acceptance of her. She was feeling heard and cared for and, in a small way, loved. She was daring to believe that she can be loved for who she really is, not for who she pretended to be. We were still a long way from breaking the fixation-on-Vince spell. But this was a small step in the right direction.

After this session ended, I thought about a Christmas present Adele's mother once gave her when she was a child. The Christmas present, wrapped in festive paper, was under the tree in a pile with all the other presents left there in the night for Adele and her brothers and sisters. Adele had told me how, in the morning she and her siblings had excitedly unwrapped their presents, tearing off the pretty paper, until she came to this one, the special mystery present she had left until last. She tore off the Christmas paper and inside she found a lump of coal wrapped in a note. The note read: 'For Adele, this lump of coal is because you have been bad'. The shock Adele felt was intense. Her mother hadn't given any of her siblings a lump of coal; Adele was the only bad one.

The email Adele had sent to Vince was the latest in a long line of 'lump of coal incidents' in her life. At the age of seven her mother sent her away to boarding school 'because I was bad'. She remembered the nights she spent lying awake in her bunk at school taking comfort from the thought that the policemen and the firemen were awake, so she wasn't entirely alone. Her ex-husband had in some ways been like Vince; she had never felt loved by him, he didn't really like intimacy, and, for the ten years of her marriage, she had constantly felt rejected.

We talked about how she was repeating the feeling of not being wanted or loved enough by her mother in all her adult relationships, including in her relationship with me in the therapy. She tried her best to be a bad client – she forgot appointments, she was late, she even tried betraying me by going to see another psychotherapist, a man, because, so she said, I had abandoned her by going on holiday and, anyway, she had wanted a man's point of view. Each time I pointed out what she was doing and made us talk about what I thought was really going on; how she was unconsciously trying to push me into playing the role of her judgemental, rejecting mother who didn't really want her. Each time she set up and acted out this scenario, I refused to play my part. But Vince was blind to the part he was playing in Adele's love script. I think Adele was obsessed with him precisely because he ignored her feelings, and constantly rejected her and refused to want her, like she believed her mother hadn't wanted her. Vince aroused in Adele the same kind of intense feelings of love that her mother had aroused all those years ago. The more he took her for granted and focussed his attention on other women, the more she was convinced she loved him because this, for Adele, was what real love felt like.

I saw Adele again some years after she had finished her therapy with me. The first thing she told me was that she was over Vince now. She then looked a little abashed and added, 'but I still occasionally feel the pull to drive past his house at night just to see if there is a light on in his window.'

Mattie's rage: A defence against intimacy

Mattie was convinced that she could not have a proper relationship; letting another person get close to her was almost unbearable, she felt so unsafe she became very angry with whoever it was and drove them away. She told herself it was because they weren't good enough. But she knew the real reason was that she was afraid of relationships.

Mattie was a successful freelance writer and copy editor in her mid-thirties. She was very thin, boyish looking, with short curly hair and big, dark, lively eyes. She was fiercely bright and deeply troubled. At the beginning of our work together we explored her childhood relationships. She said her mother was a very beautiful woman who had always been depressed, pathetic, needy. She was also endlessly demanding for material things that she expected Mattie's father to provide for her. Mattie's father was an austere, critical, remote man. She mainly remembered him escaping from the family, either by spending long hours at work or by shutting himself in his study surrounded by books. She had been very afraid of him as a child; she was still afraid of him, even now. But she loved him very much. She was the middle of the sisters and the three of them had been fiercely competitive for their parents' scant attention when they were growing up. Mattie chose the path of academic achievement, but she had never gained the praise she longed for. She vividly recalled the moments when she had been deeply hurt and humiliated by their criticism of her efforts to impress them. She even remembered proudly showing her mother a painting she had made of the whole family when she was four years old. Her mother had thrown the painting in the bin because she should have been doing her sums.

Throughout her childhood her parents had been engaged in a silent war of resentment and recrimination exacerbated by the fact that her father betrayed her mother on numerous occasions. Mattie thought that her mother's behaviour had driven her father into the arms of other women. She couldn't understand why they had stayed together. Also, she couldn't understand why she had always felt compelled to look after her mother's endless needs. She had often felt very angry with her mother when she was growing up, but she had never dared to show her anger at home.

During the early months of therapy, I often felt that Mattie was using her clever intellectual skills to block the work we were doing. I wondered if this was partly because she wanted to impress me like she longed to impress her parents – she had learnt early in life that you must be brilliant if you are to be loved. But mainly, I thought, it was her defence against revealing her unbearable feelings of vulnerability to me in the sessions. She cried when I told her this. She said later she had found this moment challenging and frightening; I was trying make her feel and she did not want to feel; she wanted to remain in her safe, angry, lonely place.

Mattie had also split off her sexuality from her feelings. She had sex every so often with a friend with whom there was no danger of love or real intimacy. She also enjoyed an occasional, strange, alienated, mutual masturbation sexual relationship with an American friend on his occasional visits to the UK. The eroticism of their sex games, free from the danger of intimacy and falling in love, attracted and excited her. These two sexual relationships went some way to satisfying her physical needs, but at the same time she was aware that emotionally she remained lonely and unfulfilled.

I asked her what it was she really wanted. She cried for a while; my question had touched her. Finally, she gazed at me with her huge, dark, sad eyes; she wanted what anybody wants, a fulfilling love relationship where the couple live together and maybe even think of starting a family. She didn't know whether she really wanted children, she was afraid to want children, she was afraid of the responsibility, the demands of children, of losing herself in her children, of becoming needy and demanding like her mother, of repeating the cold, distressing climate that had marred her own unhappy childhood. She was aware that she was using her anger and her intellect as kind of fortress – a way of defending herself against her fear of her neediness and her vulnerability – but she didn't know how to change.

But one day a change did take place. She went to a party and met a man she was attracted to, and to her amazement he was available. His name was Dominic and he had separated from his wife. The party was soon after one of our sessions when we had talked about the possibility that she might try to be more actively open with people, she might allow herself to get to know people and not to retreat into her usual hostile, defensive shell. She had fun with Dominic, they liked each other, she felt excited, they had sex, and their relationship began almost immediately.

Now when she came to see me the sessions were all about her anxieties about being in an intimate relationship, and her fear of being in love, because she had fallen in love with Dominic and he said he was in love with her. At first she found this difficult to believe; she was afraid of being in love, afraid that she would become needy and dependent on Dominic like her mother had been needy and dependent on her father. She was afraid that he couldn't possibly love this vulnerable part of her; she was convinced that she must hide it from him at all costs. Her only safe course of action was surely to hold onto her independence, to keep him at a distance, not to trust this love. Most of all she was afraid that if he really knew her, he would betray her and abandon her, like her father had betrayed her mother. She couldn't bear to think of this; if Dom behaved like her father, her hurt would be unbearable.

But the extraordinary thing was they had decided to live together, and he had moved into to her very small apartment. Her anxiety level rose sky-high. How could she maintain her distance and her independence now that they were living together? Could she trust him? Had he only moved in with her because he didn't like living alone? All the small details of her life with him were problematic: he liked to cook and eat meals together at the table; she liked to eat light snacks in the evenings on the sofa in front of the television. Now she felt heavy, bloated; she thought she was eating too much to please him. She worked from home; how could she concentrate on her work with him in the apartment? She felt jealous of his work, as if her work were not so important. How could she hold on to her identity and not lose herself in his? Even trivial things, such as how they liked to be in the mornings, were troubling her. She liked to get up early and work; mornings were her best time to concentrate on her writing. But he worked in the evenings in the theatre. He liked to lounge in bed in the mornings and have sex.

The sex was good, she said, in fact it was very good, the best sex she had ever had. I thought this was a good sign. But Mattie was even worried about enjoying the sex. She felt a compulsion to split off a part of herself and observe what was happening, as if she was sitting by the bed watching, like the scene in the film *Annie Hall* (1977), when Annie splits in two and sits on the chair by the bed observing herself having sex with Woody Allen's character. She couldn't switch off her thoughts – like, was she behaving like a sex object, or a doll, to please him? Or, was it just the sex he wanted, not her? Such thoughts hadn't bothered her with her old friend with whom she used to have sex just to satisfy their sexual needs, or when she used to play the sex games with her American guy. So why was sex with a man she was in love with different? Was it the pressure? Were the demands of love and her fear of intimacy getting in the way of her pleasure? What did I think? She very much wanted to know.

I thought that Mattie was trying to lure me into her inner world where she endlessly tried to analyse all the things that might go wrong in the relationship as a way of regaining what was for her a safe, if unhappy, distance from enjoying loving and being loved. The challenge for her was to trust the simple fact that they loved each other and enjoyed sex with each other, and to stop looking for problems everywhere. But Mattie wasn't ready for this yet. She was still afraid that the inevitable would happen; they would become like her parents and that would eventually destroy this relationship, just as these fears had corroded all her past relationships.

We embarked on many months devoting entire sessions to talking in detail about each of Mattie's fears as they arose in the relationship. The more we talked about the fears, the more the fears diminished, and gradually she dared to believe that her relationship with Dom might be different. It was already different, she even dared to believe that she was happy. Also, she was no longer angry with everyone she met. But she was still plagued by difficult feelings in social situations which she tried to avoid. I began to think she would gain more confidence in her relationships with other people generally by joining a psychotherapy group.

My therapy group was too far away from where Mattie lived, so I referred her to a long-term group being run by a close colleague of mine. Mattie and I began working through our ending slowly and carefully together. Ending therapy can bring up a new wave painful past and present feelings to do with attachment, separation, loss and fears of being abandoned. But like a separation from a loving parent, although ending therapy can be sad and painful, it's not an abandonment. It's a new beginning, bringing new opportunities for personal growth.

Some years later I contacted Mattie to ask for her permission to include her case study. She replied to say she was very happy for me to share the work with did together. She said when she read her case study it was: 'so weird to read how scared and closed up I was when we met. . . . I often share with the group what I have learnt with you. Group therapy is incredibly hard work, so different from individual therapy and terrifying at times. I am starting to acknowledge deep fears of relationship and abandonment with the group. But you were right to suggest I do this, although at times I was so upset I wanted to leave the group.

Dominic and I recently bought a flat together and moved in a few weeks ago. I'm saying this as a way of letting you know we're still together.'

5 On women, their fathers and forbidden love

The allure of unavailable objects of desire

The allure of the secret, the unobtainable and the forbidden has a powerful hold, particularly over women's sexual desires. We like to imagine that falling in love is pure and innocent, our love is untainted by our childhoods, the man we have fallen in love will certainly make a perfect husband. But as Freud, that great dasher of dreams, put it:

> The husband is almost always so to speak only a substitute, never the right man; it is another man – in typical cases the father – who has first claim on a woman's love, the husband at most takes second place.
>
> (Freud 1912)

Freud even went so far as to say, in his essay 'The Universal Tendency to Debasement in the Sphere of Love' (1912), that:

> the condition of forbiddenness in the erotic life of women is, I think, comparable to the need on the part of men to debase their sexual object.

What he is suggesting here is that, for women, the erotic attraction of forbidden, secret, and unobtainable objects of desire is universal. (Let's not get distracted by the men's need to debase their sexual objects. I shall return to this theme in Chapter 7.) Also, let's not get sidetracked by Freud's tendency to make somewhat grandiose claims that his insights are 'universal'. In my opinion there are no universal claims that can be made about the genders or their differences. However, Freud's insights do often contain tantalising nuggets of truth. But attachment theory also offers important insights into the allure of unobtainable objects of desire, particularly for women whose fathers abandoned them or died when they were children.

The father of American novelist Mary Gordon died when she was a girl. She later described the effect her close relationship with her father had on her:

> I lived at the centre of the heart of a passionate man. He loved me simply, utterly . . . certainly, I knew he was bringing me up to be no man's wife.
>
> (Secunda 1993)

It's tempting to romanticise this father-daughter relationship as special and precious. But I have seen clients whose lives have been torn apart by such an Oedipal fixation. They truly believe there is no man to equal their beloved father. Allowing themselves to love another man as much as they loved their idealised father feels impossible; unconsciously, they would be betraying their father. Attempts by the therapist to question the idealisation and normalise the father can be experienced as an attack on their core identity. Yet question it we must, if we are to address the many relationship problems that can arise as a result of an Oedipal fixation.

According to a poll conducted in 2004 by what was then the Orange Prize for Woman's Fiction, Mr Darcy was the fictional character most women would like to go on a date with. He was also the fictional character women would most like to invite to a dinner party – despite the likelihood that Mr Darcy would spend the evening gazing at the ceiling grunting with boredom or glowering rudely at the guests. One woman said the reason she chose *Pride and Prejudice* as the novel which had changed her life was 'it fanned the flames of my desire to read . . . which led to me becoming a publisher'. But then she added the downside: 'It encouraged me to fall for moody, charismatic, seemingly unattainable men, with unfortunately less happy results than for Jane Austen's heroine.'

We will never know whether Elizabeth Bennet's marriage was happy ever after – Austin portrays very few idyllic marriages in her books. But this reader perfectly encapsulates the problem.

She begins by talking about the flames of her desire to read, but she soon moves on to the flames of her sexual desire for a man like Mr Darcy. Note how she has added an important ingredient to his powers of attraction: his apparent unavailability.

Could this be why so many modern women are obsessed with Mr Darcy? By identifying with Elizabeth Bennet, they can act out the classic Oedipal fantasy – that they will be the chosen woman to save him from the dark recesses of his troubled character and set free his hidden sexual passions. In short, they will be like Elizabeth; they will transform the moody, unobtainable man into the sensitive, loving, obtainable man they secretly know he truly is beneath his gruff exterior.

What message is this Mr Darcy fixation sending to modern men? On the one hand, women say they want men who are emotionally intelligent, sensitive, flexible, who enjoy sharing equally and are fun to be with. But these same women swoon over a fictional character who is the epitome of the patriarchal male. We could throw up our hands in exasperation and conclude that some women will never learn. But I don't think it's helpful to judge women for secretly nurturing politically incorrect, forbidden erotic desires, I think it is better to try to understand where these feelings come from.

I was longing for love when, at the age of 17, I embarked on a secret love affair with a tutor at my art school. He was married and more than twice may age – an ideal substitute for my father. When I put on my psychotherapist's hat and look back at my younger self, I can see that I had found an outlet for my own unconscious forbidden desires. I had projected my idealisation of my father onto the tutor – a man whom I greatly admired but hardly knew. My fantasy even included the belief that I would one day take the place of his wife and have him all to myself. Hence the misery of guilt I felt which tapped into the guilt I felt towards my mother, whom I both loved and envied.

One of the many problems with forbidden love affairs is that they thrive on these kinds of projections. The very fact that they are secret means they exist in a parallel universe sealed off from the reality in the outside world. When fantasy meets with cold harsh reality it tends to come crashing down. I was young and needed help, but I had so boxed myself in with secrets I had no way of accessing help. Luckily, after many months of lovelorn misery, I seized the opportunity to move to a new art school and left my secret life behind.

Ellie and the Women Who Lose Themselves in Love group

Decades later, soon after I completed my training as a group psychotherapist, I had the idea of running a therapy group for women who have a pattern of unhappy and self-destructive love relationships. I think, somewhere, in the back of my mind was a distant memory of my unhappy secret love affair and the help I had sorely needed at the time.

I decided to advertise the group as a group for Women Who Lose Themselves in Love and it would run for 12 weekly sessions. I pinned flyers to various local notice boards inviting women who were interested to contact me for an individual session to talk about the possibility of them joining the group. I had no idea who would get in touch.

Ellie was wearing odd socks when she arrived for her individual session. I probably wouldn't have noticed, but a few minutes after her session began she stared down at her feet with a puzzled expression: one sock had red stripes and the other had blue spots. 'I'm sorry, I'm not deliberately trying to look funky,' she said, 'I just couldn't find a clean pair that matched.' She gave an infectious chuckle.

Ellie was 29, but she came across as more like a bubbly teenage tomboy. She was also fiercely independent; she had backpacked on her own to many remote regions of the globe. She thought she might be able to fit the group in before a walking tour in Tibet she was planning for later that year.

'When I first saw your flyer,' she said, 'I thought "losing yourself in love" sounded wet and pathetic. I hate thinking of myself like that. But the fact is, I do have a problem with hopeless love relationships. And I suppose losing myself is how I feel. It sounds awful, I know, but actually I think I am weak.'

'Travelling around the world on your own doesn't sound weak to me,' I offered, 'unless you think you are running away from something?'

'You mean like men? How ridiculous is that?' She gave a short peal of laughter.

'I don't think it's ridiculous,' I said, 'if it's how you feel.'

'It's how I feel in all relationships, like I want to run away,' she said. 'A friend asked me to dinner last week because she wanted me to meet a man, she thought I might like him. I was so scared I didn't turn up.'

I enjoyed Ellie's playful sense of humour. But I was beginning to realise that her frequent bursts of laughter were her way of defending herself against revealing painful feelings. I told her I thought the group might be an opportunity for her to explore why she felt like running away.

'I suppose so. But the thing is, I don't like groups much, I never know what to say.'

'You can listen to what the others have to say. You only need to join in if you want to. I think after a while you may find that you do want to. It's also a good opportunity to learn to talk about your feelings.'

When her session finished, I had no idea whether she would decide to join the group or not. But the next day she sent me an email telling me she was still scared of the group, but she had decided to give it go, if I would still have her.

Six women, their ages ranging from 29 to 45, were sitting in a circle waiting for the first group to begin. Ellie was the youngest and she looked terrified. The women began by talking about how nervous they had been about coming to a group to talk about love relationships. Soon they tentatively began to share their unhappy relationship stories. Out of the corner of my eye I noticed Ellie listening attentively.

'Why don't I fall in love with nice men?' mused Denise with a sad smile. She was in her mid-thirties, and still wearing her rather drab black solicitor's suit. 'I've asked myself that hundreds of times. The problem is I don't find nice men attractive. I think I see them as weak.'

'I'm attracted to smooth, handsome, James Bond types,' said Barbara, an immaculately made-up woman in her mid-forties. 'At first, you think this is the kind of man who would climb up a cliff in a raging storm for you, "All because the lady loves milk-tray!"' The group laughed. She went on to tell the group how her first husband had been a violent misogynist. She had escaped after two unhappy years, only to marry her current husband who was cold and controlling. She described herself as his trophy wife; he expected her to turn up to his work dos, but at home he completely ignored her. They hadn't had sex since her second child was born eight years ago. She suspected he was having affairs, so she decided to have an affair of her own: 'I met a wonderful man on the Internet and fell head over heels in love. The sex was amazing. But when I told him I wanted to leave my husband . . . he just disappeared. He sent me a text saying he's not good with commitment. That's why I've come to the group. I don't know what to do. He's the love of my life. I'm completely lost without him.' She buried her face in her hands and began sobbing.

The group fell silent. Heather handed her the box of tissues: 'It's not just alpha males who can be violent and controlling,' she said. She was a large, cuddly woman in her early forties. 'I'm lesbian and women can be like that too. I felt so traumatized by my ex-girlfriend's violent behavior, that for years after it ended, I was terrified of relationships. Six months ago, I fell in love with a lovely, kind woman and I'm still terrified. That's why I came to the group. I don't understand why I feel so vulnerable and insecure when I'm in love. It's almost unbearable. I'm exhausted trying to please her all the time, trying to be what I think she wants me to be. That's how I feel in all relationships. I even feel it here in the group. She stopped suddenly, as if she had said too much.

'It's good that you can talk about how you are feeling here in the group,' I said, encouragingly, 'It's an important part of the work of a therapy group.'

'I'm feeling like a fraud,' Ellie said quietly. This was the first time she had spoken in the group. 'Like I don't really belong here. I don't know how to talk about relationships. I've never had a relationship . . . well not officially,' she added, and laughed nervously.

'I have a feeling the group won't know what you mean by "not officially"', I prompted her.

Ellie took a deep breath: 'The problem is I have never told anyone about it before, except when I had my individual session.' Her voice dropped almost to a whisper. She fished tissue out of the box which Barbara had replaced on the coffee table and blew her nose loudly. 'Actually, I know I've got to tell you. It would be stupid to be here otherwise.' She took a deep breath and focussed on floor in front of her: 'I've only ever been with two men . . . The first one was when I was seventeen. He was twenty-seven and married. It lasted for about two years. He left me because he was scared his wife would find out. I was broken hearted. Then, two years later I fell in love again. This one was also married, and he had children.

She shot me a look with stricken eyes. 'I know it's terrible. I feel guilty all the time. But I'm still seeing him. We've ended it lots of times. Well, he keeps ending it. Each time I am totally heartbroken. And then he turns up again and it all starts up again. That's what I mean by 'not a proper relationship'. I've only had ones that have been hidden away like a dirty secret. I even feel bad telling you about it, as if I am betraying him. I'm not seeing him now, but only because he ended it again. I know it is me that should end it, but I can't. I really want a real relationship and children eventually. But I'm scared there is something wrong with me. I'm doomed to always choose unavailable men and end up hurt and alone.' She tried her best to laugh at herself but this time she didn't quite manage it. Instead she looked worried, vulnerable and defeated. Tears were streaming down her cheeks.'

'You're not alone,' Denise said, quietly. 'I've got a history of married men. They don't tell you until you have fallen in love with them, and then it's too late.'

I asked Ellie if she felt that she had needed to keep it a secret from the group?

'Yes,' she said, 'I'm scared of being judged, although I think I should be judged because it is so wrong.'

The group assured her that they weren't judging her, they were concerned that she had been going through this on her own for so long without telling anyone. They thought it was important that she was able to talk about it at last.

Heather said she was always afraid of being judged. 'It's just the way I am in relationships. I completely lose a sense of who I am. I have this constant, nagging feeling that I'm not good enough. I think it has something to do with how my father made me feel when I was a child. He was a big, powerful, controlling bully and I was terrified of him. All I wanted was for him to love me. I did everything to please him, but nothing worked, he never stopped criticizing me. I grew up convinced that I was completely worthless. I even thought it was my fault when he left my mother when I was ten.'

The women were engrossed in what Heather was saying, but it was time for the first session to end. Over the following weeks the theme of fathers came up in a big way.

Denise told the group how she had loved her father desperately when she was a child. 'I remember how he used to rush into our house, sweep me up in his great big hairy arms and tell me how much he adored his brown-eyed little girl.' (I noticed the group looking at Denise in her drab, black solicitor's uniform. In that moment she seemed to have transformed into the happy, brown-eyed child she used to be.) She went on to tell the group how even before her father officially split from her mother, his arrivals and departures had always been unpredictable and unexplained, leaving her in a constant state of longing for him to return.

It turned out that Ellie, Heather and Denise had all had fathers who abandoned their mothers when they were children. Ellie, who was becoming a little more vocal, told the group how her father had disappeared one day without any warning when she was seven years old: 'I thought the world had ended. I thought he had died! We didn't have any money, we had to move to a new house, and go to a different school. And then, one day, Dad turned up again, completely out of the blue. I found out later that he had run off with his secretary, but it hadn't worked out, so he had come home again. That was how it was from then on. He left us and then came back and then he left us again. My mother always took him back. I feel sorry for her now, but I remember back then thinking that Dad's leaving must be Mum's fault. I thought Mum didn't know how to love him properly. Which now seems rather unfair on Mum.' She looked at Denise: 'I adored my Dad,' she gave an ironic laugh. 'I still adore him even though he's compulsively unfaithful and a drunk.'

The group fell into a thoughtful silence.

'I've just realized that most of my men have been like my Dad,' Denise said, 'handsome, charming, funny, a little bit wild, the life and soul of the party, compulsive womanizers. I fall for the charming, funny bit, and then find myself messed around, hurt, lied to, betrayed, and on my own again. They've even been much older than me and married.' She thought for a moment. 'I'm just like my mother,' she added, angrily, 'moping at home, endlessly waiting for him to come. It's as if I am repeating what happened to her, only instead of being the wife, I'm more like one of his mistresses.'

'Both the men I fell in love with even looked like my father,' Ellie exclaimed. 'I can't believe I have never seen this before. Does this mean they were not the people I thought they were? I was projecting my Dad onto them all along?'

I thought the most striking similarity with their childhood experience of their fathers was the chaotic, emotional roller-coaster they were experiencing with the boyfriends, or in Heather's case the girlfriends. Ellie summed it up perfectly. She said the similarity for her was the longing. She used to long for her father to come home after he abandoned the family when she was a seven. It was like the desperation and the longing and the hopelessness she always felt waiting for her boyfriend to visit her, and the overwhelming love and excitement she felt when he did eventually turn up, and the awful feeling of being abandoned every time he left her and went back to his wife: 'Even this feeling I have, that if I let a man get too close to me, he will run out on me. That fits the way I was always scared my Dad was going to run out on us again.'

Heather said she understood this. She was always afraid that her girlfriends were going to leave her. Her current girlfriend was so nice and kind and constantly assured her that she loved her, but she still couldn't believe that she wasn't going to leave her.

Barbara saw the similarities between how her father made her feel and both her husbands. As a child, she had been very afraid of her father. He was a hospital consultant, his patients had treated him like God, but at home he was cold, unfeeling, judgemental and violent towards her and her mother. 'Even the love of my life (that was how she referred to the boyfriend who had recently deserted her) was somehow distant, remote, unreachable. I always had the feeling I had to save him from something very dark within himself. But I never really understood him. I think this was how I felt towards my father when I was a child, I longed for something from him I couldn't have. Love and affection, I suppose. Although I can't think why; when I think of my father now all I see is a nasty, arrogant bully.'

Heather's father had bullied and frightened her as a child. But nevertheless, she had longed for him to love her. If only she was pleasing enough, good enough, caring enough, and didn't put a foot wrong maybe he would love her. This was how she was with her girlfriend and the strain of trying to be perfect all the time was unbearable.

The revelation of the similarities between their adult love relationships and the emotional dynamics they had experienced as children with their parents was a shock to the group. The talk became fatalistic; were the patterns in their relationships doomed to repeat, was it even possible to change?

Denise became distressed. She talked about how badly her father had treated her mother, and how badly her grandfather treated her grandmother, and now the same thing was happening with her boyfriend. He had never been interested when she tried to tell him about how she was feeling or what she needed. He just put all her problems down to her being a woman and told her to get herself sorted, as if her feelings were nothing to do with him. He told her he didn't love her. So why did she do his washing for him and look after him when his wife threw him out? What was she doing? Trying to get him to need her so he would keep coming back? Was that love? Why couldn't she just turn her back on him and walk away?

The following week Denise told the group that she had ended her relationship. The group were supportive. But whilst she was talking, I had a strong feeling that she was somehow blaming me and the group for causing her to get rid of him. What good was the group if it was putting her through all this pain? She might have given up a relationship that was making her unhappy, but at least there had been some good times.

Heather told her she admired her for finding the courage to end it. She was always terrified of relationships ending, even at the beginning, she was looking for ways of defending herself against the pain of ending. She thinks this was why she finds it so hard to be herself in relationships. She was afraid if she revealed her true self she would be rejected.

Ellie said she was also afraid of revealing her true self, so she just didn't risk it. She thought if they knew who she really was, they would just see an emotional mess, or a child. She sometimes thought the answer was not to have any relationships at all. She got so completely lost in them. She was just too scared of everything. But then she ended up scared of not being able to have relationships any more. She attempted to laugh at her predicament but cried instead.

I wondered what this 'true self' was that had to be hidden away out of sight? Was it the hurt and angry part of yourself that had to be kept hidden?

Heather said for her it was a fear of being seen as worthless, because she knew she really was worthless. She always felt worthless in her father's eyes. But she also knew she was really, very angry with him. She was afraid of her anger. She didn't know what to do with it, so she held it down inside her, in her arms and in her chest, she swallowed it. Her eating disorder was about swallowing everything all the time trying to keep all her emotions down inside her. She was crying now.

I noticed that Denise was also crying. I asked her what was happening with her. She said she never felt worth anything much. She was feeling incredibly unhappy because she had ended it with her boyfriend. She also felt really annoyed with me. She hadn't felt heard by me, instead she felt I had shut her down. I said I was sorry she felt that way. But I also wondered if she had felt that way before in her life; not heard, shut down. She said she had felt like that all the time with her mother. She reached for the tissues and discovered the box was empty. I felt like a not good enough mother for bringing an almost empty tissue box.

After the group I felt that I had messed up. There had been a pervasive feeling throughout this group of not being good enough, not being lovable. I too had felt it dragging me down. I was the disappointing not good enough mother in the group. I was worried about how much it was possible to achieve in 12 weeks, whether their expectations were too high, and finally they were going to be disappointed in the group and in me. I discussed these feelings with my supervisor. (In the world of psychotherapy, a supervisor is a close colleague with whom we can share the complex and difficult feelings that often arise in therapy without breaking confidentiality.) She said she wasn't surprised. I was picking up some powerful negative projections as the parent figure in a group of women who had been disappointed, let down, judged and abused by their untrustworthy fathers. They had also blamed their mothers for driving their fathers away or not protecting them. No wonder I was feeling like another not good enough mother. Earlier in the group many of the women had complained of depression. Now they were getting in touch with their anger. That was fine. It was good if they were able to express their angry feelings with me in the group where it could be heard and contained.

The group was due to end in a few more sessions. The theme of what it meant to change was pressing. At the same time, the fear of endings and loss was also in the group. I realised the group itself had become like a love relationship; it had started out with hope, but hope was soon followed by the fear of disappointment, and the worse fear that it might end. How can you express how you really feel in a relationship, or in the group, how can you expose your true self, if you are stirred up by all these powerful feelings only to be left alone again? On the other hand, if you want to change, which is always difficult, how can you change unless you risk expressing your true self?

Heather had already begun to change her old pattern of falling in love with women who hurt her. But now she was in love with a woman who was kind to her and loved her, she was still struggling with how to receive her love, and even more difficult, to accept that she was lovable. The other women immediately insisted that Heather was lovable. They all loved her. But they also understood what Heather meant. They too found it almost impossible to believe that they were lovable.

Barbara said she had been thinking a lot about her father, and how she was afraid she might also be like him. She was afraid of being judged and evaluated, and yet she was like that too: she judged and evaluated others all the time. She also became very angry sometimes like him. Her voice dropped to a whisper: 'I hit the love of my life. I got into a temper and hit him. I can see now, that's what drove him away. I feel so ashamed.'

In the penultimate group, Heather announced that she was angry with me for ending the group: 'I still feel vulnerable all the time. I still find being in a relationship bloody hard. I'm still scared she's going to end it. I hate endings.' The other women agreed. They thought the group had helped them and they understood themselves much better. But now they were attached to their group they didn't want it to end. They looked at me accusingly. I explained that it was set up as a time-limited group with the focus on understanding their love relationships. I agreed, they had done lots of good work on themselves in the group. But I thought they would gain more, if they wanted to continue with therapy, from a long-term psychotherapy group with group members who had a variety of different problems, and with men in it. Heather and Ellie instantly declared that they would never join a group with men in it.

After 12 sessions, the group did end with tears and hugs and reproaches aimed at me. Heather and Denise opted to follow up with individual therapy. About a year later, after backpacking in Tibet, Ellie came back to see me. She was still struggling with relationships, she thought she needed more help. I risked again the suggestion that she join my long-term mixed group.

'I don't think I could to talk honestly with men in it; I would be too self-conscious, too worried about what the men think of me.'

'I think a mixed group would be a good way to help you feel more confident with men. Why don't you think about it, and let me know?'

Ellie did join the group and after a while her fears of men began to recede. Eventually she even started what she jokingly told the group was 'a proper relationship with a nice man'.

After she completed therapy, I received an email from her to tell me that she just given birth to a baby girl. In the email she said: 'I feel supported and secure for first time. And I don't think he [my partner] will run out on me! We both want to make each other happy and for the first time I can say I love you – with it not being some final last-ditch attempt to stop someone leaving me. I must say that I think the time and work I did in the groups contributed to me allowing myself to get close and show my more vulnerable side to someone – and hopefully things will continue to work out.'

6 Affectionate love and lasting sexual desire

Can we have both?

Monogamy: If prairie voles can do it, why can't we?

Freud thought there was a fundamental split in 'the sphere of love' between affectionate love on the one hand and sexual desire on the other. He concluded, somewhat gloomily, that:

> it is quite impossible to adjust the claims of the sexual instinct to the demands of civilization ... the non-satisfaction that goes with civilization is the necessary consequence of certain peculiarities which the sexual instinct has assumed under the pressure of culture.
>
> (Freud 1912)

The exception, I think, is falling in love, which is precisely the time when we do experience a powerful fusion between deep feelings of loving affection and overwhelming sexual desire. This could be the definition of romantic love. But there is a problem; we want, and expect, the feeling of falling in love, with all its heightened sexual passion, to last forever. Sadly, relationships tend to morph into what some couple counsellors refer to as 'comfortable love'. But for some couples, the dwindling of sexual desire for their partner is certainly not comfortable. The reduction in the intensity of their sexual experience, or even the complete disappearance of their sexual desire for their partner, can cause anxiety, depression, despair or resorting to the alternative, which is fulfilling sexual desires elsewhere.

Freud was not alone in thinking there is an irresolvable contradiction at the heart of our sexual relationships. Peter Fonagy, a psychoanalyst and leading proponent of attachment theory, arrived at a similar conclusion:

> The facts that sex can undoubtedly occur without attachment and that marriages without sex perhaps represent the majority of such partnerships, prove beyond doubt that these systems [affectionate love and sexual desire] are separate and most loosely coupled.
>
> (Fonagy 2001)

As we have seen, our adult attachment system is rooted in our need for a secure base and the affection, familiarity and consistency of a stable partner. This is an extension of the love and stability we needed as children from our parents or care-givers. The sexual system, in contrast, thrives on excitement, novelty, fresh stimulation or whatever it takes to bring to life our sexual feelings. Whilst it is the strength of the attachment to our familiar partner and our secure base that holds many couples together, the downside is that same familiarity and predictability can also reduce our sexual desire. One of the most often stated reasons for extramarital sex reported by the respondents to Kinsey's sexual history questionnaires was quite simply a desire for variety. One of the main obstacles to variety is the commonly held belief that marriage means lifelong monogamy.

I'm not convinced of the value of pointing to other species as a way of understanding the behaviour of modern humans. However, apparently a mere 3 percent of mammals are naturally monogamous. Prairie voles are the mammals most often cited as an example. Dr Larry Young, an American neuroscientist based at the Yerkes National Primate Research Centre in Atlanta, has conducted extensive research into the social bonding of prairie voles. He says they make perfect couples: they mate for life, they participate equally in rearing their young, and they even share nest-building duties! There is a 'monogamy chemical' called vasopressin; when prairie voles emit this magic substance, in postcoital bliss after losing their virginity, it bonds the little furry creatures in a lifelong union. But Young added a much-overlooked caveat; if a male vole happens to be wandering on his own through the prairie and he encounters a female ready to mate, he may just go ahead and mate with her. What is important, Young tells us, is that the vole always returns to the mate he has bonded with. He doesn't tell us what a female was doing all alone on the prairie when surely, she should have been safely back at home, but it seems that Young has expanded the definition of monogamy to include at least the males' occasional sexual misdemeanours!

Many humans have a more uncompromising understanding of the meaning of monogamy. For them, when two people enter into a verbal understanding or legal contract stating that now you are my girlfriend or boyfriend, official partner, husband or wife, you are no longer allowed to have sex with anyone else for as long as our relationship lasts or until death us do part. An occasional dalliance whilst wandering alone across the prairie is strictly off-limits. This is probably the most broken contract in human history, nevertheless we cling to it as an essential requirement for security and happiness in our love relationships.

It's impossible to overestimate the mess many people get themselves into over this issue. The authors of *The State of Affairs* (2004) cite an impressive number of social attitudes surveys conducted over recent decades. One of their findings, that illustrates the immense confusion in this area, was the majority of men and women, about 80 percent, say that extramarital sex is always or mostly wrong, yet many – even most – men and women admit to having had at least one affair. It's not difficult to imagine the guilt and the shame hidden behind this survey result. Another survey asked people whether they agreed or disagreed with the statements (a) companionship and affection are more important than sex in marriage or a relationship; and (b) sex is the most important part of any marriage or relationship. Over 67 percent of men and women agreed that affection and companionship were more important, whilst only 17 percent agreed that sex was more important. But, as the authors point out, 'many people practice non-monogamy secretly and shamefully, whilst continuing to accept the morality of monogamy.'

In other words, few people get through life without finding themselves at some time or other plunged into the deeply disturbing issue of infidelity, whether in their wishful daydreams, their dark suspicions, or most difficult of all, being acted out in their real-life relationships. For many people it is deeply painful to learn that their trusted partner has been unfaithful. The hurt and the anguish is acute; it's as if their whole world is falling apart. The experience of betrayal unleashes the most extreme emotions: distress, fear, rage, jealousy and for some people, obsessive thoughts about punishment and revenge.

Many straying partners also experience emotional turmoil: agonising guilt, fear of hurting their partner and their family, and panic at the prospect of losing their home if they tell their partner the truth. This is why so many people opt for secrets and lies as a way of maintaining their marriage or committed relationship, whilst at the same time pursuing their wayward sexual desires. But the price of secrets and lies, as well as the guilt and the shame, is the awful fear of being found out. And it's not only the fear of their partner finding out: the fear of being judged and shamed often extends to their family, their friends and for public figures, their reputations are in jeopardy.

In short, it is all a sorry mess. Whichever side you are on when the understanding or contract is broken, whether you see yourself as the victim of a betrayal or whether you are the betrayer, you become flooded with feelings that are so powerful and primitive it is almost impossible to think straight. But when your future and the future of your partner and children are at stake, there are few times in life when it is more essential to think straight.

What strikes me about this dichotomy between comfortable affection and a more diminished sexual desire on the one hand and re-awakened passionate sexual desire on the other hand, is just how impossible many of us would find it to choose one over the other. Most of us want loving, affectionate companionship *and* to be sexually passionate and fulfilled with the same partner in a stable long-term relationship. I'm certainly not saying this aspiration is impossible to achieve. There are couples who do remain faithful and sexually fulfilled throughout their long relationship. But there are also many couples who don't manage it.

Some couples work through the pain, the hurt and the lies in couple therapy. They come to see the infidelity that has brought them to therapy as a symptom of problems they have failed to address in their relationship. When did they stop listening to each other? When did demands of work and the needs of children take over completely? What about all the simmering resentments they have brushed under the carpet? How come they keep pushing sex to the bottom of the to-do list, or it gets lost altogether? Rather than see the infidelity as a reason to separate, they realise it is a wake-up call to revive and enliven their commitment to each other.

There are also couples who decide that for them the problem is monogamy itself. They know they love each other, they value their commitment to each other, but they also want, or need, for whatever reason, the freedom to have sexual encounters with other people. But they don't want their relationship to be contaminated by secrecy and lies. These couples opt for mutually agreed non-monogamy as the way forward. For some couples this decision is driven by necessity. One person in a couple may no longer want to engage sexually and be content that their partner finds sexual fulfilment elsewhere. Or one partner may develop a sexually debilitating disability or long-term illness and not want their partner to be deprived of sexual fulfilment. Or one partner may be bisexual, or they want to explore sexual inclinations that are different from their partner's. Or a couple may decide that non-monogamy is preferable to breaking up the family home and causing their children distress. Some couples simply decide that they don't believe in monogamy.

I think for non-monogamy to work, honesty with each other is essential. It's also important to agree together on a set of boundaries. For instance, some couples agree that their home is off-limits for casual sexual encounters. Others decide to try sharing their non-monogamy experiences by attending partner-swapping events or inviting a third person for a threesome to revive their sexual excitement together. Most couples who opt for non-monogamy say that the sexual encounters with others must be purely for sex, without emotional entanglements. I think trying to legislate against emotions, such as falling in love with someone new, is a tough one, and for many people it just doesn't work. In any event, couples need to know themselves very well if they opt for non-monogamy. If it's a guilt-free ploy for one person in the couple to play the field whilst their partner feels increasingly lonely, neglected and unhappy, or if either partner tends to be jealous, making a non-monogamy agreement may just be a way of avoiding the inevitability of breaking up.

In short, I don't believe there are any simple right or wrong answers when we are confronted with the monogamy problem and issues of infidelity and betrayal. The way forward depends on the people involved, their specific circumstances, their psychological dispositions and the stage they have reached in life. But I do know that thinking together with a psychotherapist, counsellor or couple therapist in a safe, confidential space can help us to understand what is happening to us, to manage the intense emotions that flood us at such times and to think about why they appear so impossible to resolve. Therapy can also help us to work through the many dilemmas and choices facing us and to find a way forward.

Douglas's very disturbing infatuation

Douglas, a tall, bald, slightly overweight Scotsman, was an architect in his late forties. Despite his attempts to look smart in his business suit and designer glasses, he always managed to appear somewhat dishevelled, as if he were in a never-ending struggle to tame a part of himself that was threatening to get out of control. This struggle, it turned out, could also be a description of why he had come to see me.

He arrived with a list of reasons he wanted therapy. Top of his list was anxiety, trouble sleeping and incipient depression. He had had a depressive episode in his past before he met his partner, Sarah, and he was scared it may be coming back. Second, he had a feeling there was something wrong with his life; he wasn't fulfilling his potential, although his architectural business was doing fine. Third was his mother: he wasn't sure why she was on the list, but since his father died some years earlier, she was always talking about dying. He didn't know why; her doctor didn't seem to think there was anything wrong with her. But it was upsetting. Fourth, for the past year he had been deeply troubled by a romantic infatuation with a woman called Juliet. Fifth – he had forgotten what the fifth was – oh yes, he wanted to be tougher. He had always wanted to be tougher.

I asked what he meant by 'tougher'.

Less of a people-pleaser, he supposed, more like his elder brother. His brother had always been his mother's favourite, the brilliant one, the golden boy who could do no wrong in his mother's eyes. His brother had bullied Douglas horribly when they were children. Douglas had also felt that he was a disappointment to his father. He was the family clown, the lazy one, the not good enough child. He also had younger sisters and wondered if part of this not good enough feeling was because he had never been able to get enough attention.

I asked about Juliet, the object of his disturbing infatuation. He said she was an interior designer in her forties with whom he worked occasionally. He described her as the polar opposite of his partner, Sarah. Juliet, he said, was fascinating, mysterious and beguiling. Sarah, a busy lawyer, was practical, straightforward, sensible, a wonderful companion and an excellent mother to their twins, a boy and a girl, who were both at university now. He paused for a moment and took a deep breath. Sarah knew he had a friend at work called Juliet, he continued, they had always chatted away to each other about everything that was going on in their lives. But he hadn't told Sarah about his infatuation. He had never lied to Sarah. He just didn't tell her what she didn't need to know. There was nothing to tell anyway, he hadn't had sex with Juliet – except in his fantasies. They had never even kissed, not a real romantic kiss; he hugged her when they met and kissed her on the cheeks in the continental way, nothing more. Juliet flirted outrageously and loved to be surrounded by adoring men. That was all he was to Juliet, he was sure, just another adoring male lusting after her. But the smell of her perfume and just the slight brush of her lips on his cheek was totally intoxicating. Each time he saw her all he could think about was seeing her again. He gazed at me helplessly with a boyish grin on his face: 'Juliet is like the archetypal Hollywood goddess, gorgeous and unobtainable. I know that, but it doesn't stop me thinking about her, all the time.'

I had a feeling that Douglas would happily have entertained me with stories about his infatuation with Juliet for the rest of his therapy, but I wanted to hear more about his relationship with Sarah. He was silent for a minute. He then said carefully: 'I would prefer to keep my relationship with Sarah off-limits. It's very important to me that therapy doesn't make me want to leave her. I've thought about it, of course, but I know I don't want our relationship to end.' He looked at me suspiciously.

I knew he was feeling threatened by therapy and wanted to reassure him. But it is difficult to fence off a part of our life as off-limits in therapy. Stuff comes up in therapy, as if of its own accord, despite whatever we do to police our unconscious and keep it under wraps. However, I decided to wait until he brought the subject of Sarah up again.

The story of Douglas's sexual liaisons with Liliana, a night cleaner in his office, just tumbled out one day. He looked at me wide-eyed as if he could hardly believe it himself. Liliana was a large Portuguese woman. She was even older than him, in her late fifties. She was not at all the kind of woman he would have thought he would have sex with, yet they had had sex quite a few times, on the sofa in his office at work. It started one night when they were alone in the office. He was watching her empty the waste paper bins and it occurred to him to ask her about her life. To his amazement, she told him that she hadn't had sex with her husband for ten years and this made her very sad. She said, 'I am a woman, I need the sex.' The next thing he knew they were having sex on his sofa. They had absolutely nothing in common, but the sex was incredible: 'She actually said to me: You have a very beautiful body', he said, imitating her thick Portuguese accent and glancing ruefully down at his girth. He glanced at me bashfully: 'You're smiling.'

He was right, I was smiling. 'I'm sorry,' I said, 'it was something about the way you told your story that made me smile.'

He grinned: 'I am glad you are smiling. I thought I would be too ashamed to talk about it, but now it feels good to have told you. It's all a bit mad though, isn't it? I'm romantically infatuated with a woman I have never even kissed properly, although since telling you about Juliet my fantasies about her seem to have gone away. I am fucking the office cleaner. And I love my wife. I don't know what I would do if Sarah found out.' He paused for a moment and added, 'Actually it's the thought of Sarah finding out that terrifies me.'

'I can't help wondering how you feel about your sex life with Sarah,' I said carefully, recalling his anxiety about therapy upsetting his relationship. I didn't want to sound too intrusive.

He struggled with his reply. It was easier to talk about his romantic infatuation with Juliet or sex with Liliana than it was to tell me about sex with Sarah. They didn't have sex as frequently as they used to, he said. But he thought that was normal after 20 years of marriage. It's just not very exciting anymore, but it's fine. Their relationship worked because of their companionship; sex was never the most important thing. When they did have sex, it was usually at the weekend at his instigation. He paused. I could tell by his frown that he was finding this next thing hard to say: 'Sarah is a very practical person and she works really hard. She's too tired to make love when we go to bed at night. She masturbates sometimes instead. She says it helps her get to sleep.'

'How does that make you feel?'

He hesitated: 'I think it's ok if it helps her sleep. She's an independent woman, a feminist, and very grown up about things like masturbation.'

'That sounds very understanding of you. But I was wondering more about your feelings, if Sarah is masturbating to help her sleep rather than wanting sex with you?'

'I suppose I feel a bit shut out. Although when we do have sex, she says it's good. It's just that at night it's too much effort, and she comes more quickly when she makes herself come.'

'You feel shut out.'

'Something like that. I feel unnecessary, superfluous to requirements, a bit unwanted. I don't know. I think I try not to have feelings about it.'

'So, Sarah masturbates and goes to sleep, and you are left lying awake unable to sleep?'

'The problem is Sarah likes to come quickly because she's got a busy work schedule and for me sex with Sarah takes longer . . . I don't get as excited as I used to, I don't desire her so much in that way.' He trailed into silence and looked upset. 'I can't believe I said that. I wish I hadn't. I feel awful, disloyal. Somehow actually saying all this out loud makes it sound more real. This is why I didn't want to talk about Sarah, I don't want to rock the boat.' He removed his glasses and began furiously rubbing his eyes. 'I love Sarah. Although sometimes I think I don't even know what love means anymore. But I do know for sure that I need her, and I don't want to end our relationship.'

But sex was rocking the boat whether Douglas wanted it to or not. In our sessions he brimmed with vitality when he talked about his infatuation with his goddess, Juliet, or sex on his office sofa with Liliana. Whereas in his relationship with Sarah he felt superfluous, inadequate, not good enough to satisfy her needs.

He hated criticising Sarah in our sessions; it made him feel disloyal, guilty and anxious. But in a later session he told me he had been thinking about the type of women who appear in his sexual fantasies. They were usually big, soft women. He said the fantasy felt quite primitive; he longed to be held by a big, soft woman with large breasts and cuddled, touched and massaged like a baby. Sarah was small and thin, not very tactile, not into cuddles and hugs. And he was never sure that she really desired him. Sex was always at his instigation. He liked being desired. I thought of Liliana, who he described as a very large woman. And I thought of his mother, who would have appeared big and soft to him when as a small boy he envied his brother and younger sisters for getting all her attention and her cuddles whilst he felt overlooked.

The following week, soon after he arrived for his session, he said he was worried because he had been thinking that he might not be giving me what I want, he wasn't being a good enough patient, I wasn't satisfied with him. I wasn't surprised. These or similar insecurities about how I felt about him frequently popped up in our sessions in various guises. I felt sure they originated in his relationship with his mother and he was unconsciously transferring them onto me, and onto Sarah. I had also been wondering if I appeared in his fantasies. If so, I doubted they were sexual – I'm a small woman, nothing like his big, buxom Liliana. It's always a difficult question to ask, but I decided to go ahead.

'I've been thinking about your fantasies, and wondering if I appear in them, or how you see me?'

He grinned and said: 'No, no sexual fantasies about you, I'm afraid. I see you more as a mother. But a benign authority figure, not a disapproving martyr-ish woman like my mother who always leaves me with the feeling that I'm not doing enough to look after her.'

'Like you arrived here today with the feeling that I'm not satisfied with you because you are not giving me what I want in therapy? But what if we turned this around? What if you were annoyed with me because I wasn't giving you what you want? I'm the one who is not good enough. Would you tell me?'

'Probably not. I would just stop coming to see you.'

'That would mean you would be stuck with your feelings of being annoyed or angry or unsatisfied with me. And if we couldn't talk about it, you would be depriving our relationship of the possibility of change. Is this what is happening with your mother and with Sarah?'

He admitted the following week that he didn't enjoy this session. He didn't feel unburdened like he usually does after therapy. He felt hectored and he didn't like it when I hectored him. Sarah hectored him. He rebelled sometimes, but in a childlike way, like mending his bicycle in the sitting room when she was away. He knew he was a chronic conflict avoider, not at work, professionally he was okay with conflict. But he quickly backed down if there was danger of any conflict with Sarah, his mother – or me, he added cautiously. His safe place was that of the accepting stoic, the nice guy. But he knew he wasn't really accepting, he was just left feeling frustrated and resentful. He wanted to be tougher, but he was afraid of rejection.

At the beginning of his therapy he had said that he was afraid of his mother dying, but once he began talking about death his own fears came tumbling out: fears of cliff edges, flying, car accidents, apocalyptic catastrophes, prostate cancer. Familiar fears, but also for Douglas, exacerbated by some traumatic deaths in his family history which fuelled his pervading sense of anxiety. I also wondered if his recent preoccupation with death was about his fear of losing his potency, and maybe a feeling that a part of him was dying or was not fully alive. His romantic infatuation with Juliet and sex with Liliana were ways of keeping alive his vitality and potency and warding off these existential fears. But it was Sarah who gave him his sense of security, she was the one who grounded him and gave his life structure and meaning. No wonder he was terrified of losing her.

Towards the end of Douglas's therapy, he told me he had been to visit to his father's grave. He mopped away tears as he told me how he had fled from the grave and then felt terrible because he had betrayed his father by running away when all he ever wanted was his father to be proud of him. I was very moved as I listened to him and, at the end of the session, I told him that I felt concerned for him. He immediately tried to reassure me that he would be fine. I pointed out that he had slipped into his familiar mode of feeling that he had to look after me, when I had just wanted him to know that I felt moved by his story. He burst into tears.

Having your feelings taken seriously and being heard is what touches us most deeply. It's good to learn not only how old familiar feelings have a way of inserting themselves into our current relationships, but also to discover that it is possible to let go of these feelings. It is possible to change.

When we met for our final session, Douglas told me he now felt less anxious, less resentful, and he was standing up for himself more with his mother and with Sarah. Also, his sex life with Sarah had improved.

'I'm not sure quite how it happened, but I feel different now, I feel stronger, tougher. I always wanted to be tougher,' he smiled.

'Yes, I remember,' I said 'Wasn't that your fifth reason for coming to therapy?'

It's not difficult to see how Douglas was caught in the conflict between his need for affectionate love and security and his wayward sexual fantasies and desires, which Freud believed was a universal affliction in civilised society. But knowing, intellectually, that we are all, to a greater or lesser extent, caught in this paradox, doesn't make the feelings of anxiety, guilt and shame go away. Psychotherapy doesn't have solutions to universal moral dilemmas. But it does provide a place where confusing and deeply troubling contradictory feelings and impulses can be safely shared.

And difficult feelings that have been denied, or too shameful to talk about, can at last be given the airtime they need and even, hopefully, put to rest.

Dulcie and the allure of the rejecting object of desire

Dulcie had known about her husband's affairs for 12 years, maybe longer. She could hardly believe that she had put up with it for so long. She knew she couldn't go on like this, but her fear of change was extreme. She felt very ashamed, as if there was something wrong with her.

Dulcie was an artist in her late forties. She had been married to Philip for 25 years. At first, she had thought it was just one affair. Philip's business had frequently taken him abroad, and she believed him when he said he would never do it again. She loved him, and she very much wanted their children to have a proper family life. But now the children had left home, and she was finally gaining some real success with her work, she had two exhibitions in the pipeline – it was the rest of her life she was worried about.

The problem was, Philip never stopped having affairs, lots of them, and it turned out that it had been that way for most of their marriage. She paused for a moment, as if hearing herself tell me this was still shocking, even though she had known for a long time. She wondered if she had turned a blind eye because she couldn't face the truth. She paused again, and then ploughed on, she needed to get it all out. She said she felt hurt, horribly confused and most of all, scared. The trust had gone. They had seen a couple counsellor about a year ago, but it was useless; he lied to the counsellor. It was this endless stream of lies that upset her most. That, and his inconsistency.

'What kind of lies?' I asked.

'Mainly about the other women. He says he wants to be faithful, I believe him, and then it becomes obvious nothing's changed. I don't understand it. It's not as if we don't have sex. We have never stopped having sex. I like sex. I don't much like the way he always wants me to dress up in sexy underwear like a porn star, but I go along with it if it pleases him. But still he lies about the other women. He told me once there was no connection between him desiring other women and not enjoying sex with me, and if I could only accept that everything would be fine. But I feel as if I don't know who he is anymore. Maybe I never really knew him.'

'I'm constantly afraid of making the wrong decision,' she continued. 'I don't want to tell him to leave, tear the family apart, and then regret it. But how can I spend the rest my life with a liar and a manipulator? Or is the problem with me? A friend told me it takes two to make a divorce, whatever that means. Another friend was so shocked when I told her about Philip's behaviour that now she just keeps telling me he's a bastard and I should leave him. That makes me feel even worse. I wish I hadn't told her. The problem is I can't focus on my work. I can't sleep. I'm constantly preoccupied by what is going on with Philip. I feel very close to panic. I know this can't go on. I have to make a decision. But I can't. What do you think I should do?'

'Dulcie, apart from the fact that I don't know what you should do, my role isn't to tell you what to do. I'm here to help you understand yourself better until you know, yourself, what is best for you. But it will take time,' I said.

I think she was relieved. Unlike her friends, I wasn't pressing her to make a life-changing decision before she was ready.

She gazed sadly at the flames licking around the coals in my gas fire. 'I like your fire,' she said.

'I like it too,' I said.

'I would like to have a fire like that in my studio. Until then, I will just have to come and enjoy your fire with you.'

'That sounds like a good plan,' I said.

We embarked on what turned out to be a long course of therapy, our conversations shifting between her childhood and her marriage.

'My mother never loved me,' she said, bluntly, when I asked about her childhood. 'I remember as a child longing for her to love me. A part of me still longs for it, which is strange. She's an old lady now, you would think I would have given up. She was always a cold, critical, manipulative woman with very high expectations of all of us. I don't think she even knew how to love. When I was ill in bed as a child, I was left alone for hours on end, crying, wanting my mother to come and comfort me, but she could never be bothered. My father came instead. I think he knew she was neglecting me, and he did his best to compensate, which was maybe why we developed a special bond.'

She fell silent. I had a feeling she was thinking about her father. I asked her to tell me more about him.

She smiled, sadly. 'He was one of those old-fashioned men who finds it almost impossible to express feelings, he was never comfortable with cuddles or hugs. But he was a good, kind man with strong moral principles. He would never have dreamed of being disloyal to my mother. I found out years later that she had been disloyal to him. I wasn't surprised, she always made it perfectly clear that he was a disappointment to her. I could feel my father's hurt, even when I was a little girl. But I always knew that he loved me. And I loved him. I felt completely alone and abandoned when he died a few years ago.'

I thought it was interesting that the man she had chosen to marry appeared to be the opposite of her father. I mentioned this to her in a later session and she agreed. She met Philip when she was in her mid-twenties. She had had quite a few boyfriends, but it was Philip she fell head over heels in love with. She had been fascinated by him, she still was fascinated by him; he was exciting, interesting, dynamic. He had also been the most fun, and she liked having fun.

'One of the first things he told me about himself was "I am a man with monstrous appetites"'. She burst into a peal of laughter. 'I suppose I should have seen that as a warning. But I remember I was intrigued and excited. I even think it was partly his badness that attracted me'. She shook her head, as if marvelling at her younger self. 'Now I just see him as greedy and selfish.'

'Perhaps, although you loved your father, a part of you found his goodness constraining and stifling?' I suggested. 'You knew somehow that you needed something different in your life, to break free to enable you grow. After all, you wanted to be an artist. Maybe you wanted to learn to be bad?'

She frowned. She had known how to be bad when she was young, she insisted. She had flirted outrageously, played with her boyfriends' feelings, led them on and dropped them quite callously. She had been quite attractive in those days and not afraid to use her sexual power.

I said I thought she was still very attractive, I could easily imagine that men would see her as a powerful woman.

She batted my comment away. 'I don't feel as if I have any power. Anyway, that was a long time ago. I've changed. Also, I wouldn't like to be like that again. I don't like women who wield sexual power in that flirtatious, callous way.'

'Power isn't always bad,' I said. 'Feeling your own power can be important.' She was frowning; I could sense that she disagreed with me. But I also had a feeling there was something important about this conversation. I tried again: 'By locating all the badness in Philip, in a way maybe you are giving him all the power. Maybe, to be free, you need to take back some of this badness and this power for yourself?'

After the session, I felt as if I had been on shaky ground when I had talked about power. I had a disturbing feeling that now she thought I was bad, and I wondered if she disapproved of me?

The following week she told me she had been thinking a lot about this session. She had realised that, apart from those few years when she was a student, she had always been very afraid of being bad, particularly when she was a child. She had never been able to tell lies, and she usually trusted people, whereas Philip was the opposite: he didn't trust anyone. 'He particularly doesn't trust you. You are his latest bugbear. He's convinced you are on a mission to make me leave him. He refers to you as: "that woman you go to see"'. She laughed, she liked it that his feathers were ruffled by her coming to see me.

One day she told me that Philip had had an angry outburst: 'We were in the kitchen. He was pouring himself a drink. I think he was already a bit drunk. Anyway, he suddenly lost it. He announced that if the truth was really what I wanted, then he would give it to me. He couldn't give up other women. He didn't see why he should give up other women. They make his life more interesting.

He likes sex with me, *and* he likes sex with other women. Sex is one of his greatest pleasures. Whereas lots of things make me happy, like painting. I can sit alone in a field all day and be perfectly happy. He's not like me. He hates being alone. Anyway, he finally said what he wanted. He wants me to agree to an open marriage.' She stopped speaking and stared at me. 'I can't imagine having an open marriage. It doesn't make any sense to me. Why be married at all? I know if I have sex with another man it would mean I would no longer want sex with Philip, and that would be the end. Loyalty and honesty are an intrinsic part of my identity, they are very important to me, that's just who I am.'

'Like your father?'

'Yes, I am like my father. And I loved my father for his loyalty and honesty.'

'It sounds like Philip is saying sex with other women as well as with you is intrinsic to his identity,' I suggested. 'The question is, can you accept him as he is?'

'I really don't know,' she said, 'But I do know I can't live with an open marriage.'

Dulcie was constantly bewildered by Philip's inconsistency. A few weeks later, her hopes were raised again. Philip told her he had changed his mind about an open marriage. Now he wanted to be faithful. He was thinking about seeing a therapist for sex addiction: 'I don't know anything about sex addiction,' she said in exasperation, 'but I told him I thought it would be a good idea for him to see a therapist. I just don't know what to believe. Does he really want to change? Or is this another ploy to manipulate me whilst he goes back to seeing his other women in secret? What do you think?'

I had wondered if Philip's behaviour was what's sometimes called Don Juan syndrome – a compulsive need to seduce women, not just one, but lots of women (see page 134, Chapter 7). But during Dulcie's sessions I frequently caught myself falling into the trap of joining her in trying to analyse Philip, as if by proxy. I had to remind us both that it was Dulcie's therapy, and her unconscious motives were what we needed to focus on, not Philip's. The important question was, why was Dulcie endlessly preoccupied with trying to understand Philip, as if one day she would find the magic key to getting him to change?

As a child Dulcie had been similarly preoccupied with her mother. She remembered thinking that if she knew why her mother didn't love her, she could find a way of making her mother love her. Her strategy, to gain her mother's love, had been to be a very good and undemanding child. Even if she had hurt herself, or if she was distressed, which she often was, she never went to her mother for help or comfort; she knew her mother wouldn't be interested in her hurt. She wondered if her marriage with Philip had lasted because she wasn't very demanding, she protested occasionally, she made it clear she was unhappy, but finally she had always gone along with whatever Philip wanted.

I found myself thinking that maybe, unconsciously, she was projecting her mother onto Philip. She was still the undemanding, self-sufficient child who didn't make demands or ask for what she needed. 'What is it you would really like from Philip?' I asked.

Her reply was instant: 'More than anything I would like him to share his feelings with me. I want to feel closer to him, I feel as if I don't know who he really is.'

When she got home, she told him what she had told me. It backfired. He flew into a huge rage, slamming his fists on the table and shouting at her that he was telling her what his true feelings were. He needed sex, he liked it, sex with other women was no big deal. He didn't care about the women. Sex with her, with the other women, sex with himself, it was all just sex! It was the only relief he could get from anxiety. That WAS his feeling!

The force of his rage had shocked and frightened her. But this was also the moment when she realised that her feelings towards him were changing. The man she saw now was lost and insecure, and incapable of showing any vulnerability or weakness, instead he became angry. He was frequently drunk, afraid of ageing and terrified of dying. At work he was important; the boss surrounded by his admiring employees and adoring secretaries. At home he was constantly restless, in need of ego boosts to enable him to feel alive. She was ashamed to admit it, but she preferred her old image of him as powerful and confident, even as a Lothario, he was more attractive. The man she saw in front of her now was diminished; his secret world, where he hung around in bars and picked up women, was a dark, seedy, pathetic place. She no longer knew how she felt about him.

She was also beginning to finally accept that he wasn't going to change, he hadn't changed in 25 years, he was clearly flagging up to her that he was not going to give up his many affairs for her. The question was whether she can accept him like he really is and be reasonably content with their companionship, which was important to her – he was a good companion, he was fun and funny, and she enjoyed their conversations when he wasn't drunk or shouting at her – or should she leave him?

Soon after his outburst of rage, Philip went away on one of his many business trips. This time he was away for two months. At first Dulcie said she was relieved he had gone, she had space to breathe, she was getting on with her work, seeing her friends, and she was happy. Until, one day she received an email from him. She said she knew that he was with another woman; she could tell from the tone of the email. He also mentioned the possibility of divorce. They had talked about divorce before, but when she read his email she was pitched into a full-scale panic. Could this really be the end of their marriage? She spent the night alone, curled up like a foetus hugging herself, crying and shaking. The state she was in was so terrible, she had thought she couldn't survive it.

When she came for her session a few days later, she told me she recognised the terror from long ago; it was her fear of being abandoned by her mother and left utterly alone. Terrible as this feeling was, it helped us understand why, despite her strong conviction that she could not be happy with Philip as he was, she was seized by a paralysis when it came to the finality of leaving him. In the past, she had been fine when he was away because she always knew he was eventually coming home to her. The thought of being abandoned and alone forever was too much for her to bear.

But Dulcie was changing. She was growing stronger and clearer about what she wanted. She met a man in an art gallery one day and arrived for her session brimming with excitement. His name was Giles. He was single, extremely attractive, interesting, very intelligent, and they had already slept together. Their sexual compatibility was unlike anything she had experienced before. She had fallen in love. The problem was Philip was coming home and he now was saying he didn't want a divorce, he wanted to make their marriage work. But after meeting Giles, she couldn't imagine having sex with Philip, she said: 'It would feel like she was betraying Giles'.

Soon her divorce proceedings were underway. Ideally, this would have been the beginning of Dulcie's new life with Giles. But as is so often the case in real life, things turned out to be more complicated. Giles was an artist and a recluse. Often, after spending a few days with her, he would take flight and resist all contact with her, sometimes for weeks. Dulcie would never know if or when she would see him again. Just as she was giving up hope, he would get back in touch and they would meet, spend a few passionate nights together, and then Giles would again retreat into his defensive shell, leaving Dulcie feeling confused, neglected and abandoned.

I had a sinking feeling when she told me about his behaviour. I didn't doubt Dulcie's conviction that their love was mutual, but he had never lived with a woman and, by the sound of it, something about a committed relationship frightened him. But how could she turn her back on him? She was in love, and for the first time for a long time she felt alive, sexually desired and stimulated creatively. Her painting was progressing in leaps and bounds.

Whereas in the early part of her therapy Dulcie had spent hours trying to understand Phillip, she was now telling me about everything she and Giles had said and done together. She was desperately trying to understand why he kept withdrawing from her into his reclusive shell. Could Giles's behaviour be explained by his lifelong difficult relationship with his domineering mother? Had his mother made him afraid of women? Maybe, deep down, Giles hated women, like he hated his mother? Again, Dulcie was in a constant state of trying to work out what she was doing wrong to cause Giles's neglect, and each time he withdrew from her she was afraid that this time he really had abandoned her. The only thing that alleviated her fear and her loneliness was when he got back in touch. She knew everything was not all right – far from it. But the relief she felt when she heard his voice on the phone or saw him waiting on her doorstep when she arrived home was like a drug that brought her back to life.

I agreed, the relief she felt when she saw him again was like drug addiction. Giles's unpredictable behaviour was constantly bouncing her between the highs of their passionate encounters and the lows when she was in a state of anticipation, longing and acute anxiety, never knowing when or if she was going to see him again. Possibly it was an unconscious defence mechanism on his part, but it did show a worrying lack of empathy for her feelings. Whenever she tried talking to him about her feelings, and the basic reassurance and stability she needed in their relationship, he would refuse to respond or even to hear her.

Now that her marriage with Philip was over, she was lonely. She badly wanted the contentment and companionship of a committed loving relationship. She even tried breaking up with Giles by joining an online dating site. She half-heartedly began a few new relationships, but she soon became bored; none of the men was as fascinating, interesting, or sexually fulfilling as Giles. She was always deeply ashamed when she told me she was back with Giles; she was afraid I would be disappointed or disapprove of her. I didn't feel disapproving, but I was concerned. I wanted her to be happy, and Giles's unpredictable, avoidant behaviour appeared to be making her more unhappy than happy.

One day, Dulcie arrived for her therapy session and presented me with the most difficult question I have ever been asked by a client.

She said: 'After all the work we have done together, I really do understand the similarity between my childhood longing for my mother's love, the love she could never give me, and my tendency repeat the dynamic with men who neglect me like my mother neglected me. But this doesn't explain why Giles and I are so sexually perfect together. He feels it too, I know he does. Does this mean I am facing a horrible choice? On the one hand, I stick with what I have; the most wonderful sex with Giles, but he is so afraid of his feelings he doesn't know how to be in a relationship and I am constantly plunged back into the neglected place by his disappearances. On the other hand, I could try to end my relationship with Giles, and find a man who can at least give me the reassurance, security and companionship I want. But what if I never find another relationship as sexually fulfilling?'

We sat looking at each other in silence for a while. Eventually, I said that I didn't have the answer. But I was holding on to the hope that one day she would find a new partner who could give her both: the sexual passion and the comfort of a secure, affectionate, loving relationship. But, for many people, not just her, the desire for both may remain an unobtainable dream.

Annie's yearning for 'proper sex'

For some people, the shame of having been unfaithful is unbearable. The suffering is made even worse if there is no one they can tell; they are entirely alone with their secret. This was the reason why Annie came to see me.

Annie was in her late thirties. She had been married to Hugh for seven years. She loved her work as a piano teacher. She also gave occasional concerts and played for a local choir. Hugh was an accountant, and they owned their own home, which they had renovated together. She and Hugh were like best friends; they were incredibly compatible and agreed about most things. She knew she should be happy, but for some time now she had been becoming increasingly irritable and depressed. She said she knew what the problem was, but it was very difficult to talk about. Tears began streaming down her cheeks. She grabbed tissues by the handful, said she was sorry and grabbed more tissues. It was as if after years of holding back her tears the dam had finally burst. When she was finally able to speak, she told me her story.

About six months ago she had gone completely off the rails and done something unforgivable. She picked up a man in a bar and had sex with him. She couldn't believe she had done such a sleazy thing. If Hugh ever found out it would be terrible. At the beginning of their relationship Hugh had told her about the time when he found out that his ex-girlfriend had betrayed him and how for him sexual betrayal was totally unforgiveable. The man Annie had sex with had been much younger than her and she didn't even like him. But it was as if her body had taken over, this man had awakened something in her and she wanted sex with him desperately. Afterwards, she had ended it and told him never to text or email her again. But she still felt like a woman obsessed; she couldn't get sex with him out of her mind, she couldn't stop thinking about sex, about wanting 'proper sex'. Since ending it with him she had become very depressed and deeply ashamed of what she had done. Also, Hugh had noticed the change in her, although of course he had no idea what was wrong. How could he know? He trusted her.

She finished her story. I could feel her relief that at last she had been able to tell someone her 'shameful secret'. I was also aware that she was probably thinking that I was judging her as harshly as she was judging herself.

I wasn't judging her, of course. I was puzzled.

'Annie, what do you mean by "proper sex"?'

'Penetration', she said immediately, 'I need penetration to feel like a proper woman, I long to feel a man come inside me. But for Hugh sex is all about foreplay, sex toys, vibrators, anything ... except he won't come inside me. None of the other stuff means anything to me if he won't come inside me.'

She went on to tell me that she could count on the fingers of one hand the times they had had 'proper sex'. Even at the beginning of their relationship their sex play had consisted mainly of mutual masturbation because this was how Hugh liked it. It wasn't that Annie didn't enjoy sex that way. But for her sex wasn't only about having orgasms. She just wanted him to come inside her sometimes at least. At first, she thought it was because Hugh was afraid she would get pregnant. He knew she wanted a baby and although he wasn't exactly enthusiastic, he said he was okay with it if that was what she wanted. But after a while she thought maybe he didn't want a baby and couldn't admit it, so she decided to go back on contraception to see if that helped. 'I got fitted with a cap, but I've hardly used it. The damn thing just sits there in the bathroom cupboard mocking me. That was years ago. Now we hardly have sex at all, not even the foreplay kind. Hugh doesn't seem to mind whether we have sex or not. But the awful thing is, now I don't want sex with him anymore. It's worse than that; I can't bear the thought of sex with him. I've developed an aversion. Sex with my husband feels unthinkable. It's as if we share our lives like best friends or brother and sister. I love him, and I know he loves me. He's devoted to me. He trusts me. That's what's so awful, how could I have done this terrible thing to him. He would be devastated if he found out. I feel guilty, sordid, disloyal and scared.'

The problem of Annie's guilt about her betrayal was important, but it also seemed to me that her shame kept diverting us away from the sexual problem.

'Annie, I understand that you feel very guilty,' I said. 'And I know it's important that we talk about it. But I am also wondering what's going on with Hugh. Have you tried talking to him about your sexual feelings and asking him about why he doesn't want to come inside you?'

'I've tried lots of times, but Hugh has always hated talking about sex. He gets embarrassed. And now I've given up. I'm also scared that if I try talking to him, he will be able to see in my eyes that I've betrayed him. Because he doesn't suspect anything, I haven't had to tell any lies so far. I've always been a terrible liar. I panic. I blush horribly, and I feel as if my nose must be growing huge and will give me away, like Pinocchio. Pinocchio was my favourite film when I was a child.' She managed a weak smile and then frowned. 'There's another thing; I'm scared that if I try talking to Hugh, I will have to have sex with him again and now I've got this aversion to him. How could I possibly tell him that?'

No wonder she was in a state of panic and anxiety. She refused to even think about couple therapy with Hugh, so they could work together on their sexual problems. Apart from the fact that Hugh would never agree to therapy, she was also terrified by the prospect of Hugh finding out that she had betrayed him. She was convinced that if Hugh knew about her disloyalty it would hurt him so deeply it would destroy their marriage. She was also terrified by the thought of splitting up with Hugh and losing her secure home and all the good things about their marriage. She couldn't bear the panic and anxiety of being unfaithful again but the prospect of never having 'proper sex' was equally unbearable. She was going around and around in circles with no way out.

The root of Annie's terror about losing Hugh became more apparent when we talked about her childhood. Annie's father had deserted the family when Annie was a toddler. Annie hardly saw him throughout her childhood, although he occasionally got in touch. After he left, Annie's mother decided that she had had enough of men, from now on it would be her and Annie, just the two of them. Annie adored her mother and for as long as she could remember she was afraid of losing her too. Her mother, who was older than all her school friends' mothers, had become seriously ill when Annie was five and she could remember being very afraid that her mother was going to die, and she would be left alone with no one to look after her. Luckily her mother didn't die and, in the village where they lived for the first ten years of Annie's life, she felt loved and secure, she had friends at school and all the people in their village knew her. But then her world fell apart; she and her mother moved to London. Also, her mother was drinking too much, much too much. As a teenager Annie rebelled, she was angry with her mother and even more afraid of losing her now she could see that the drink was killing her. When she was 20 the dreaded thing happened; her mother died. Annie was left alone in the world.

The more we talked about Annie's relationship with Hugh, the more it appeared that Hugh had taken the place her mother had once played in her life. They were each other's best friends, it was just the two of them together in the world and Annie's sense of security had become entirely dependent on him. No wonder she felt such an extreme panic at the thought of losing him; this was how she had felt as a child about the prospect of losing her mother. Her act of disloyalty, which was perhaps also a rebellion and an expression of her anger with Hugh which she could not express in their relationship, was exacerbating her panic and her guilt. She had grown up in a world where disloyalty and betrayal were the worst of sins; her mother had never forgiven her father for leaving her for another woman, just as Annie was convinced that Hugh would never forgive her for what she had done.

We spent many hours exploring how Annie's current unbearable feelings of panic, anxiety and guilt were certainly partly a result of her relationship with Hugh, but these feelings were also fuelled by her childhood with her mother. Nevertheless, the sexual problem remained; she wanted sex, but she still felt an aversion to sex with Hugh. What to do?

The big question we had been unable to answer was why was Hugh so resistant to full-blown sexual intercourse? She had wondered if he was gay and in denial about his sexuality. But other than his resistance to penetration, there were no signs that he might be gay. Could it be that he simply preferred the stimulation of sex toys and mutual masturbation? We discussed the possibility that he was suffering from an acute form of performance anxiety. Or maybe he was in the grips of a primitive, unconscious fear of being swallowed up by a woman. If so, I could imagine that such a fear would be extremely difficult for him to talk about. Whatever the cause, I thought it might help if Hugh, or the two of them together, saw a psychosexual therapist. But Annie continued to be adamant that Hugh would never see a therapist.

However, as Annie began to feel less overwhelmed by her childhood fears, she also felt stronger and more convinced that whatever the problems in her relationship with Hugh, she knew absolutely that she did not want their marriage to end. She loved him too much and didn't want to lose him. In the end she worked out her own solution. She and Hugh had decided to go on a long, exotic trip abroad. She said she was determined to use this break in their usual routine to reignite their relationship and their sex life.

I wrote to Annie a few years later to ask for her permission to use her story. She sent me a prompt reply and an update, 'for the sake of accuracy'. She told me she and Hugh had been on several wonderful trips together and had more planned. She was also much happier, and more at ease with things as they had grown closer and their marriage had become stronger. She felt lucky that she had been able to save things in time. On the other hand, they hadn't had any discussions about sex: 'Somehow, it's as though we have decided to put that away completely . . . I am unable to contemplate sex in any form now and wonder whether in fact the real problem has always been mine. I sometimes feel terribly guilty and sad for him as well as for me. I don't know what the answer can be, short of doing my best as a wife in every other respect. And I know that he is doing his best to be loving and more easy-going which is making a big difference. Perhaps in time the intimacy will come back.'

I felt sad when I read Annie's email. It's nice to have an unequivocal happy ever after ending. But there are rarely neat resolutions in life or in therapy. Annie had decided that she had gone as far as she wanted to go in therapy for the time being. And she is far from alone with an unresolved sexual problem. It's not unusual for couples to find themselves in the situation where they no longer have sexual intimacy, but somehow, they settle with what is often an unspoken agreement that the love, comfort, companionship and security they both gain from their relationship is more important to them than sexual fulfilment.

On the other hand, in the future Annie and Hugh may come to see their marriage and their sex life differently. Life is an ongoing, unpredictable and complex process. Stuff happens; we all inevitably grow and change. Whatever stage we have reached in life, the decisions we make can only be what feels right in the here and now.

7 On pornography, prostitutes and sex addiction

Why are some men attracted to sexually debased women?

In 1912 Freud published an essay with the provocative title 'On the Universal Tendency to Debasement in the Sphere of Love'. The essay is complicated, and I think it's a bit of a muddle. But as usual with Freud, it contains some fascinating insights.

Freud begins his essay by discussing a sexual problem that he said was one of the most common complaints to arise in his consulting room. His patients described the problem as 'a feeling of an obstacle inside him, the sensation of a counter-will which successfully interferes with his conscious intentions.' In other words, his patients were describing a feeling of being sexually blocked, as if a powerful unconscious force was standing in the way. There are many reasons why some men become impotent and some women don't like sex. But these men appeared to be saying there was something preventing them becoming sexually aroused when they thought they ought to want sex with their wives. They were able to perform sexually, but the sex didn't give them much pleasure. When it came to sex with women whom they thought they shouldn't enjoy sex with, it was quite another story. The problem was, these were women from the lower classes: servants or prostitutes. Why should this be? This was the question that interested Freud, and also interests me.

The year 1912 was very different from the modern, high-tech, sexually permissive 21st century. Gender roles and class hierarchies were far more clearly defined. There was a strictly enforced division between the immaculately dressed, respectable mothers, wives and unmarried daughters who inhabited the drawing rooms of upper-class and middle-class households and the female servants below stairs, women from the lower classes and the prostitutes who stalked the streets in the poor areas of town or were hidden in the sexual underworld. However, even in our modern society many of these divisions remain; we still have a split between the domestic arena inhabited by the mothers, wives and girlfriends, and the many women who make a living from the sex industry: porn stars, lap dancers, strippers and prostitutes.

Nowadays, for many wives and girlfriends, acting the part of a sex object, dressing up and performing sex like a prostitute, lap dancer or porn star, as a way of pleasing men, has become a routine part of sex play. And men often expect women to serve them in this way as proof that they are sexy and good in bed. This kind of playacting isn't necessarily exploitative. When it comes to sex, women also like to throw off their inhibitions, go a bit wild, feel free and have fun. However, some women say they feel objectified and almost detached during sex; the expectation that they dress up and perform like the classic male fantasies of sexy schoolgirls, femme fatales or porn stars acts as a barrier to the kind of loving intimacy they really want. Also, there is a big difference between willingly playing the part of a debased sexual object and the unwanted experience of being coerced, used and abused sexually. The many scandals which precipitated the #MeToo movement are just one example of how widespread the modern debasement of women remains.

To get back to the question that interested Freud, and that interests me, why is it that some men find that they can gain full sexual gratification only from prostitutes or women who are demeaned, cheapened, or beneath them in some way? As usual, Freud turned to the Oedipus complex for an explanation. If something about the wife or official sexual partner reminds the man (or his libido) of his mother, or maybe a sister, the problem may be an unconscious repulsion by the slightest hint of incest. Or, as we saw in the previous chapter, the kind of affectionate love the man feels for his wife or partner in his familiar domestic surroundings may over time cease to arouse his sexual desires. This contradiction in the sexual system, between familiar affection and sexual novelty, leads some men to Internet pornography and even prostitutes for fresh sexual stimulation.

Another reason, according to Freud, that some men were attracted to debased women in the sexual underworld was that their respect for women inhibited them sexually. They were too embarrassed or ashamed fully to let themselves go sexually with a woman they loved, admired and respected. They idealised her femininity in such a way that she was too perfect or too fragile for sex, as if she needs to be protected from men's base sexual desires. In other words, the problem lay in an irresolvable conflict between their idealised image of femininity and the primitive, animal nature of the sex act itself. Visiting prostitutes was a way of protecting the idealised women in civilised society from this shameful part of themselves. This sounds to me like a somewhat coy Victorian explanation. Or it could be a sign of Freud's own tendency to overlook issues of power and powerlessness in gender relations. Some men are simply afraid of women's sexual power and what can be unbearable feelings of vulnerability, loss of control and powerlessness aroused by real intimacy.

There are many different reasons for visiting prostitutes. Some men visit the brothel to safely act out their sexual fantasies, such as a masochistic craving to be treated like a supplicant child by an all-powerful mother substitute. The prostitute is asked to play the part of a school matron or dominatrix, to walk on them or whip them into submission. Some men prefer sex with a prostitute because it is free from intimacy; the financial transaction means there are no demands on them to perform or even to please the woman. The brothel can also be a place where men can freely express the part of themselves that nurtures deeply hostile feelings towards women. They need to be in a position of sexual power over a woman whom they pay to be degraded and demeaned. Whatever the reason, paying a prostitute means the man is ultimately in control: he is paying her to do his bidding.

However, there will always be men – perhaps the majority – who have no desire to pay for sex. These are men who routinely debase and degrade any women they have sex with by treating her as a sex object who exists solely for their sexual gratification. For such men, debasing women is so routine and normal they don't even realise they are doing it. They are imitating men in their peer group, and often they have grown up in households where their fathers routinely denigrated or abused their mothers.

Conversely, there will always be men – perhaps many men – who repress their true sexual natures and quietly accept that their sexual lives will not bring them much satisfaction, or they lose interest in sex altogether.

Whilst Freud's main interest in his essay was men's tendency to desire debased women, he briefly made what I think is a fascinating observation about gender differences. He noticed that, unlike men, most women didn't sexually desire men whom they saw as debased or beneath them in some way, and they didn't have a need to debase men sexually to excite their own sexual arousal. The force driving many women's eroticism was a passionate desire for sexual partners who were idealised, unavailable or forbidden (see page 89, Chapter 5).

I think that hidden – or not so hidden – behind our modern veneer of gender equality these different erotic tendencies of men and of women are still common, not for all men and women, but for many. I also think that these different erotic tendencies might offer a profound insight into a significant difference between the genders with implications that go far beyond the erotic to cast light on some deeply entrenched problems in relations between the sexes generally (see Chapter 9).

Why do some people become addicted to sex?

Every civilisation throughout history has had pornography and prostitutes, and there have always been compulsive and addictive behaviours associated with sex: 'the painful condition of feeling controlled by one's sexual desires and compelled to act on them has been described as far back in time as the third century by St Augustine' (Hall 2013). The game changer for modern culture has been the advent of the Internet. It has vastly increased the easy accessibility, the temptations and the opportunities for every kind of sexual stimulation, whether it's surfing for pornography or prostitutes, or using mobile phone swipe apps, like Tinder or Grindr, as virtual market places for nearby and available potential sexual partners. Apart from the sites for gay men and lesbians, the pornography on display in the heterosexual underworld is mostly controlled by men and aimed at fulfilling male fantasies, and most of the objects of desire are female.

Sex addiction is an obsessive preoccupation with sexual gratification that feels out of control. It is not restricted to men, there are some women are also addicted to sex, but it is far more common in men. At the time of writing, sex addiction is still not officially recognised in the DSM (*Diagnostic and Statistical Manual of Mental Disorders*). Nevertheless, increasing numbers of desperate clients are seeking help for what has become for them an addiction to sex. For some men their sex addiction is focussed on multiple and hugely costly visits to prostitutes. Other men spend hours and hours secretly masturbating whilst watching pornography online. These clients mainly come for individual help. But I have also seen couples who are desperate for help when a wife or girlfriend has been shocked and, in some cases, become distraught when she has discovered the true nature of her partner's secret sex life.

Sex addiction can take a variety of forms. For some men their compulsion involves seducing unusually vast numbers of sexual partners. This is behaviour is sometimes called the Don Juan syndrome after the legendary, fictional Spanish libertine who devoted his life to the pursuit, seduction and conquest of multiple women. The author Jane Austen wrote in one of her letters, after a trip to the theatre where she saw the character of Don Juan in a play: 'I have seen nobody on the stage who has been a more interesting Character than that compound of Cruelty and Lust.' She's not alone in her fascination with the character of the libertine. The spectre of a seasoned seducer who apparently adores women, but whose lust is also driven by a callous disregard or cruelty towards the feelings of the women he seduces, is a powerful combination. Superficially, the narcissistic libertine appears to be having a great time, freed from empathy or concern for his prey and the usual social constraints placed on sexuality. Some powerful and narcissistic libertines, such as some of the men outed by the #MeToo movement, probably were having a great time until the women found the courage to tell their stories.

But there are also men who are deeply distressed by their obsessive-compulsive behaviour and their complicated and contradictory feelings about women. They sincerely believe they love and respect women, so why do they feel in the grips of what amounts to an addiction to sex, particularly if the objects of their desire are women who work in the sex industry, many of whom are exploited?

Paula Hall is the author of *Understanding and Treating Sex Addiction* (2013). As research for her book, Hall, a psychotherapist who specialises in sex addiction, conducted a UK survey of people, mainly heterosexual men, who suffered from sex addiction. From the 350 people who responded to her questionnaire, she was able to see some common threads. There is no simple answer to the question of why some people become addicted to sex, but it is rather a combination of causes. One in three respondents to her questionnaire cited easy access to sexual opportunities in puberty or earlier as a major factor. This cause is particularly disturbing given the easy access children and young people now have to on-line pornography at an age when their brains are still forming. We don't yet know how this will impact on their sexual lives in the future. Also, sex addicts, in common with people who are addicted to drugs and alcohol, often have a history of distressing childhood experiences: loss, painful separations from loved ones or emotional, physical or sexual abuse. Sex, substance abuse or a combination of the two is an attempt to manage or self-medicate distressing feelings. The problem then escalates to a point where the addiction itself rapidly becomes the cause of distress, which requires more sex, drugs or alcohol to treat the distress – and so the vicious cycle is set in motion.

Sixty percent of people in Hall's survey described their family background as strict and controlling. Any rebellious behaviour had to be acted out in secret. Seventy-seven percent said they grew up in a family where either the emotions expressed were extreme and frightening to a child, or no emotions at all were expressed, instead there was a climate of cold silence. As Hall puts it, these children grew up without a 'model of how to healthily experience anger, sadness, frustration, loneliness, loss and so on.' Sex became their way of managing and soothing all their painful emotions. Fifty-two percent said they had been made to feel bad and worthless as children as a result of excessive criticism, hostile silence or both. They had learned to defend themselves by being secretive from an early age and shame was a dominant feeling for them as they were growing up. Forty-one percent began using pornography before the age of 12. For them, 'lone, secretive, shame filled sex became the norm'. A massive 64 percent said they felt 'lonely, isolated or different in adolescence'.

A common scar of trauma, whether the cause is emotional, physical or sexual abuse, is anger; anger at the perpetrator, anger at the person who failed to protect you and anger with yourself for being a victim. But anger is experienced as a difficult and dangerous emotion to manage: if it gets out of control, it threatens to expose secrets and lies and result in catastrophe. It is safer to numb any feelings of anger, fear and acute anxiety with sex. This habit of using sex to numb feelings fuels the addiction. Sadly, for many the sex addiction blights their lives with feelings of immense guilt, shame, unhappiness, loneliness, depression and despair. Lars was one of these people.

Lars's addiction to pornography and prostitutes

Lars, in his mid-thirties, worked for an independent production company making TV programmes. My first impression, when he strolled into my consulting room, was of a man who was confident and completely at home in his own skin. He was tall, slim, blond and casually dressed in jeans and T-shirt. I watched him as he seemed to drink in the room, the books, the pictures, the fireplace. Finally, he smiled and said he liked my room, it felt warm and inviting. I liked him immediately, although I made a mental note to be careful; I can be a sucker for charm, which isn't necessarily helpful for clients in therapy.

He told me he had been in therapy once before; he and his ex-girlfriend had been to couple therapy for about six months: 'The problem was I lied all the way through the sessions and

Ester, my girlfriend, ended up dumping me anyway. Ester was, is, everything I've ever wanted in a woman; great company, brilliantly intelligent, beautiful, successful. I don't blame her for dumping me. I know it was my fault. I was behaving badly, and I felt guilty for behaving badly, which made me behave even more badly.' He gave a sudden burst of mirthless laughter. 'I was gutted when she dumped me. I still feel gutted, although I know I've been a shit. I didn't deserve her.'

'What did you lie about?' I asked.

'Sex', he said, 'my porn habit mainly', he paused for a moment as if deciding whether to continue, and then he added: 'I was also spending a fortune on prostitutes.'

He was studying my face. I could feel him searching for a reaction, maybe disapproval or disgust.

'Okay, go on'. I smiled, encouraging him to continue. If a psychotherapist is judgemental, she is in the wrong profession.

'Ester didn't know', he continued. 'She probably would have been okay with the porn, that's sort of normal. But I couldn't imagine telling her about the prostitutes. She would have been horrified. I suppose the truth is, I lied selfishly, because I didn't want to lose her. That's why I had to lie to the couple therapist. Don't worry, I promise not to lie to you. This time the therapy is for real. I know I need help to sort myself out. I'm in a real mess. Really, I promise not to lie to you.'

'That's good to hear. Lying to your therapist doesn't make much sense,' I said. 'But sometimes it's difficult to know what the truth is. I get it that you lied because you didn't want to lose Ester. But I'm wondering if the lying was also because you didn't want to give up the prostitutes? Have you given up prostitutes?'

'I'm trying to. I want to. I really want to. But not much success so far, I'm afraid. That's why I need your help. It's completely mad. I can't afford it for a start. I dread to think how much money I've spent on prostitutes over the years, a fortune.' He paused. 'It's not easy for me to talk about this,' he said, quietly. 'I've never told anyone before. Even on my way here today, I was trying to work out how I could tell you my problem was obsessive-compulsions without telling you the compulsion was seeing prostitutes.'

'You know I'm not an addiction specialist. There are groups for sex addiction, and there's the twelve-step programme.'

'I know, but I don't want to join a group. I feel safer here with you. I really want to give it a go.'

I was worried. Working with sex addiction is notoriously difficult. But there was something about Lars, and the urgency in his tone, that touched me.

Over the next few sessions Lars told me his story. He had discovered telephone sex when he was 14. He said he had been a skinny, spotty kid, terrified of girls and scared of sex. He couldn't remember how he knew about telephone sex. He thought he probably saw it advertised in one of the porn magazines he had hidden away in his bedroom. He couldn't remember the first time he had phoned, although he must have been scared. 'I was convinced there was something wrong with me, I was different from the other kids, I was sexually inadequate in some way. I couldn't even kiss a real girl, let alone have real sex. It would have felt like betrayal.'

That word 'betrayal' surprised me. 'Why a betrayal?' I asked.

He seemed as puzzled as me about why that word 'betrayal' had popped into his mind. He finally decided that the problem was the atmosphere in his house. Sex didn't exist: it was completely off the radar, his parents never talked about sex and he couldn't imagine even going out with a girl let alone taking a girl home. However, he did eventually manage to lose his virginity a few years later at university when he was 18 – in the normal way, he assured me, with a real girlfriend and not a prostitute. But he remembered feeling at the time as if he was exploiting the girl somehow; he felt guilty afterwards maybe because she said she was in love with him and he knew he was going to leave her. Whatever the reason, the sex with this girl wasn't great. By then he was hooked on telephone sex and pornography, and he knew already what he really wanted. A few weeks later he visited his first prostitute.

Since then his sex life had been split between what he called 'official sex' with girlfriends and 'secret sex' – which was either masturbation using pornography, or sex with prostitutes. The problem with sex with girlfriends had always been that he found it hard to relax. He felt an intense pressure to perform. It was important for him to please his girlfriend and he was worried about premature ejaculation; he thought he came too quickly. With prostitutes he felt free from the pressure to perform, maybe because she was the one who was performing, and he was paying.

'I always felt tawdry and guilty and afterwards. I hate the hypocrisy of it. I hate it that by going to a prostitute I am participating in the exploitation of women. That's why I always try to be extra nice to them, to make up for fact that I'm exploiting them. I kid myself that really they like me because I am nicer to them than their other clients, and I am really helping them because they need the money.' He gave a short bitter laugh, as if he couldn't believe he had said that. He then looked at me helplessly: 'Look, I know how pathetic this sounds. But at least it's the truth. . . . But there is something else too.' He faltered and looked shame-faced. He wanted to tell me, and he was trying hard to be honest for the sake of the therapy, but he found this next bit even more embarrassing.

He took a deep breath: 'At first I asked the prostitutes for normal penetrative sex. But later I got the courage, if you can call it courage, to ask for what I really wanted, hand-jobs. Well, not just a hand-job, there's also the fantasy. I begin by telling her the fantasy, then she has to talk me through the fantasy while she's giving me the hand-job.' He looked at me steadily: 'You want to know the fantasy, don't you?'

Well, yes, of course I did.

'God, this is embarrassing . . . humiliating. You realise I have never told anyone this before, don't you? Well, except the prostitutes.' He took another deep breath. 'Okay, here goes; the fantasy is that she has to tell me in detail about the best sex she's ever had with a big stud with a great big cock.'

I was puzzled: 'So you don't want to be the stud?'

'No,' he said. 'I don't want her to pretend I am the stud. I want her to talk me through the most amazing sex she ever had with the stud. He must be someone else, a man with a great big prick. That's it.'

'Is this something you wish you could witness in reality?' I asked.

'Absolutely not. It's the girl telling me about it I want.'

'So, you are turned on by a story you are excluded from?'

'I suppose so, in a way,' he said, doubtfully. 'But it's me she's focussing on when she's giving me the hand-job and telling me the story.'

Lars said the ritual begins the moment he starts searching the Internet for a prostitute. The excitement and anticipation build steadily until he arrives at the brothel and the girl gives him the hand-job whilst she talks him through his fantasy scenario. When it's over, he feels a moment of immense relief. 'But it doesn't last long,' he added with a wry laugh, 'because it's always followed by an overwhelming feeling of self-disgust.'

He thought for a moment before he added a final piece to the puzzle – each time the prostitute must be a different girl and she must be a class below him, not at all like his middle-class parents or his sophisticated girlfriends. The prostitutes he chose all had similar physical characteristics. They looked like a couple of the older girls at his school. He vividly recalled these two girls: 'They were the ultimate unobtainable objects of desire. I remember the day I came across them giggling together behind the bike sheds. They showed me a picture they were admiring in a porn magazine. The picture was of a classic male porn star with a truly enormous prick. Great picture to show a skinny, spotty, under-developed, little kid who is deeply ashamed of his sexual feelings.'

'What did you feel?'

'I don't remember feeling anything. Sad maybe, inadequate. I was probably already thinking about finding a phone and doing telephone sex.'

For years Lars's ritual with the prostitutes had been the same. He didn't want variations. It was only through the precise enactment of each step in the ritual that he found relief from his intense feelings of anxiety and dread. The pursuit of relief from his acute anxiety appeared to be a significant driving force behind all this. But what was the root cause of his anxiety?

Lars was an only child. He assumed he must have been close to his mother when he was very small, but he found it hard to find the words to describe their relationship when he was growing up: 'It wasn't so much that she was cold, distant, maybe, with my Dad, and in a way with me. I was always worried about her health, she's been ill off and on for as long as I can remember. She was probably depressed, married to a man like my Dad. He was a seriously angry man. He's not so bad now, I guess age has mellowed him a bit. But when I was growing up, his rages were completely irrational, totally mad, endless sarcasm, criticising everything and everybody as if he hated the entire world and everybody in it. He constantly attacked, criticised, judged and belittled me. I was terrified of him. My mother probably was too. She never once stood up for me.'

'So, your father was the big prick in your house?' I suggested.

'I prefer to think of him as a big bully,' Lars said, dryly. He narrowed his eyes and looked at me suspiciously. 'I think I know where you are going with this. But the stud in my fantasy is like a big dick from a porno movie, he's not like anyone I know, and certainly not remotely like my father. I cannot imagine my parents ever having sex, although I suppose they must have done it once.'

'I was wondering if you had ever seen them having sex, maybe when you were very little?'

Lars frowns, but I can see he's interested; he looks alert. 'I remember going into their bedroom once when I was little, about four. I don't remember why – maybe I had had a bad dream and wanted my mother to comfort me. Anyway, my father was on top of my mother and she was moaning weirdly. I was scared he was hurting her. But I don't recall feeling anything about it, just the event.'

Lars dismissed the memory; if he didn't feel anything it can't have been important. I was thinking that it wasn't surprising that he couldn't recall feeling anything; after all, what was a frightened little four-year-old boy to make of the alarming thing that was going on in his parents' bed that night? Given that he was already terrified by his father's rages and worried about his mother's fragility and frequent illnesses, any disturbing sexual excitement or arousal he may have experienced combined with fears of the possible violence or violation that his father may have been inflicting on his mother would have stirred up feelings that were far too overwhelming for a four-year-old to contemplate – safer to forget the whole episode, banish it to his unconscious and go back to bed.

In the next session Lars told me he hated going home to his empty flat. Since Ester had left him, he had really let the place go. It was uncared for, unloved, a mess and dark because he couldn't be bothered to get new light bulbs.

'Sounds like your flat is a mirror of how you feel,' I said.

'I suppose so. I really messed up with Ester. I miss her. For the first three months we were in love and happy. Ester adored me and mothered me, and the sex was good. But she started having to go away for work trips. I felt abandoned and went back to prostitutes. When she came home, I used to give her a really hard time. I was moody, angry, depressed, jealous and nasty.'

'You became like your Dad?'

He stared at me: 'Not nearly as bad as him. But that's why she left me. She got fed up. I don't blame her.' He was quiet, trying not to cry.

'What was your bedroom like when you were a child?'

'It was like a hotel room. Lonely. I was a lonely kid.'

'Can you remember being in that bedroom?'

'I remember being in there at night in the dark. I was afraid of the dark. It didn't feel like a safe place. I was scared that my Dad might come in at any moment and shout at me in a mad rage because I hadn't done my homework properly. I was in a permanent state of anxiety and dread throughout my childhood. He made me feel worthless, as if I could be stamped out at any moment, as if I was nothing. That's the feeling I remember from most from my childhood, feeling like nothing.'

We sat in silence for a while.

'It sounds to me as if your father emasculated you,' I said.

Lars stared at me in shocked silence.

At the end of the session, just as he was leaving, he turned to me and said that he had found my suggestion that he had been emasculated very hard to bear: 'That hurt,' he said, 'but the reason it hurt was because it is true. See you next week.'

I made a note to return to it next week. But the following week Lars arrived in a state of heightened anxiety. He said he had made a big mistake; he told his mother he was seeing a therapist: 'I told her in confidence. I made her promise to keep it a secret from Dad. But she told him. Now she's trying to manipulate a situation to get me to talk to Dad. I should have known not to trust her. She's been doing this all my life, manipulating things to placate Dad. Everything has always revolved around him, and her needs. My needs never mattered. Even when she abandoned us, she wasn't thinking about what it would be like for me left alone with him.'

'She abandoned you?'

'She left my Dad when I was about thirteen or fourteen. I got home from school and discovered that she was gone. I found a letter from her in my bedroom. I can't remember what was in the letter, just the dread of how my Dad was going to react when he got home. How could she have left me alone with him? One thing I remember was thinking of how I could use this to my advantage. I was secretly in love with this girl at school. I thought if I told this girl my mother had abandoned me, she would feel sorry for me and fall in love with me. I think I really wanted her to give me a cuddle. Anyway, it didn't work, the girl wasn't interested. That's when I first started doing telephone sex. My mother was gone, the house was empty when I got home. The sex worker couldn't see me, she was just a voice talking dirty to me at the other end of the line, she didn't know she was talking to a spotty little kid. On the phone I could be anyone.'

'How long was your mother gone for?' I asked.

'I can't remember. I can't even remember the day she came home. I guess her bid for freedom hadn't worked. But I remember the day my father received an enormous phone bill. My grandmother was visiting from Sweden. My Dad marched into the dining room where we were having breakfast and denounced me: "This disgusting son of ours has been doing telephone sex!" or something like that. It was an itemised bill. Of course, he had phoned the number to find out who I had been calling and got a shock. He was like the worst kind of ham actor, waving the phone bill around in the air like a mad person. I remember burning with shame. How could he do that in front of my grandmother? The humiliation was awful. I ran. The next thing I remember is trying to work out how I was going to do telephone sex now I had been found out. But I was a resourceful kid, I soon found ways round it.'

'You make it sound as if, even at the age of thirteen or fourteen, you were some kind of cool, calculating manipulator,' I said. 'But all I can see is a lonely, unhappy child who went to the girl at school because you were looking for someone to mother you. Maybe that's also what you wanted from the women on the other end of the phone sex lines?'

'Maybe. But I think I was manipulative. Or maybe it's more accurate to say I was a failed manipulator.' He grinned.

As usual, Lars found it hard to feel anything about his childhood, or to hear me when I said I felt touched by his story.

'Did either of your parents ever talk to you about why you were doing telephone sex?' I asked.

'God no, that would have been unbearable.'

'If you were the father of a fourteen-year-old and you found out he was doing whatever the modern equivalent is.'

'Webcam sex,' Lars said, flatly.

'Okay, so your fourteen-year-old child is hooking up with a sex worker doing webcam sex on his computer, would you think it was a good idea to talk to him about it?'

'Yes of course I would. But after the phone bill incident neither of them ever mentioned it to me again. I suppose if they couldn't talk to each other, they couldn't talk to me either, about anything except school work. They were both obsessed with exam results. Nothing else mattered to them. I felt like a constant failure, until I got into university, they were pleased about that.'

Lars usually started his sessions with the number of days since he had last relapsed. As the therapy progressed the numbers grew. He was doing well. He had even cleaned up his flat and brought new light bulbs. But on day 60 he got home to find a message from his father on his answerphone. His father said he was prepared to meet Lars anytime, anywhere and talk about anything Lars wanted to talk about.'He sounded almost reasonable, apart from making a bad joke about even talking psycho-babble if that was what I wanted.'

'What do you feel about meeting him?'

'I don't know. I'm still scared of him, that's the problem. I can't imagine telling him how I really feel.'

'What would you like to say to him?'

Lars thought for a while:'I could ask him why he was always so angry?'

'I suppose you could. It's a bit vague. What would you say to him if he was here with us now?'

'Get the fuck out of my therapy session, you bastard!' Lars instantly shot back.

I smiled, 'Okay.'

'Why were you such a shit father?' Lars added, he was getting in the mood.

'That's better.'

He suddenly looked deflated:'You realise I couldn't say anything to him without him twisting it to his advantage.'

'Maybe what matters more is you telling him what you feel. Not what he does with it,' I suggested.

Lars decided he wasn't ready to talk to his father, not about feelings anyway. He was convinced the inevitable outcome of talking to his father would be catastrophic. It would mean the end of their relationship. His mother would suffer, and he would feel responsible and unbearably guilty. He preferred to stick to his usual strategy of keeping conversations calm and neutral. I wondered if, unconsciously, Lars's fear of standing up to his father was also a fear of taking the lid off a life-time of his own bottled up rage. Maybe that was the catastrophe he dreaded. What if, like Oedipus, he killed his father?

Christmas arrived, and the inevitable happened. The row between Lars and his father rapidly escalated until it was in danger of becoming a physical fight. At that moment, Lars backed off and smoothed things over in his usual conciliatory way. But something had changed between them. Lars had suddenly realised that he was physically bigger and stronger than his father. His father was getting old and he seemed shrunken and almost lost. Lars felt sorry for him. He realised that, despite everything, his father loved him in a kind of twisted way, and he loved his father.

However, his struggle with his addiction continued. We wondered if maybe the Big Prick in his fantasy was a kind of gift to the prostitute? By getting her to feign sexual excitement with the Big Prick he was ensuring that he wasn't a disappointment to her. I wondered if maybe the excitement he felt when the prostitute told him about having sex with the Big Prick was an indication of an unacknowledged part of him that was bisexual? But he was adamant that he no desire to have a threesome, at least not with another man. I began to think that the meaning of the fantasy wasn't the important thing. What mattered was the fact that a masturbation fantasy had first imprinted itself on his mind when he was a vulnerable, pubescent teenager, a time when his brain was still forming. That was when the girls at school had taunted him with the pornographic pictures of the stud with the enormous prick. He had turned to telephone sex as a way of alleviating intense feelings of loneliness, abandonment, dread and anxiety, and somehow an association, with the image of the big prick and a woman's voice talking to him to assist the excitement of masturbation, had got stuck. The ritual of a prostitute talking him through the fantasy whilst she masturbated him, was added later when he saw the prostitutes in person. And now, whenever anything in his life triggered acute anxiety, his automatic response was to act out the entire ritual to regain control of his emotions and finally, briefly, find a kind of relief. But this was invariably followed by feelings of self-disgust, worthlessness and a kind of dark self-destructive pessimism with one saving grace, which was, as Lars put it: 'At least it felt real'. For Lars, 'feeling real' was the thing, even if that 'real feeling' was entirely self-destructive and threatened to bring his world crashing down.

After the fight with his father their relationship improved. It wasn't long before he fell in deeply in love with Gale. He met her in the old-fashioned way at a friend's dinner party. Gale was beautiful, bright, emotionally intelligent and sexually adventurous. They shared sexual fantasies and pornography. They moved in together and Gale made his flat feel like home again.

But let's not jump to happy ever after just yet. Lars was happy with Gale, he was no longer seeing prostitutes, and sex with Gale was great. But Gale had a demanding job that often took her abroad. The old abandonment issue returned. Lars also began to miss his sessions with me and text lame excuses at the last minute. When he did turn up, he would tell me about his new 'happy self'. Or he would relate some traumatic memories or interesting dreams. But I had a feeling he was trying to please me by telling me the kind of stories therapists like to hear. He was also trying to seduce me with compliments. He praised me for being a good therapist. He even ended one session by saying excitedly that he was in love me, probably because of some pearl of wisdom I had dropped into the session. But somehow it didn't feel quite real.

I told him, after he had missed two sessions in a row, that I thought he was trying sabotage the therapy. 'I also think you are trying to sabotage your chance of happiness with Gale,' I added. 'And Gale sounds like really good news to me. I think this is what you do in relationships. First you idealise the relationship, with Ester, with me, with Gale, but then you feel in danger of losing the part of yourself you think is worthless and resort to your familiar pattern of secrets and lies.'

'You mean, I'm not just a wanker?'

I ignored his attempt at a joke, 'I don't believe you are worthless, if that's what you mean. I think you are struggling with the part of you that is still that traumatised child. The fantasy, the prostitutes, it's all a manifestation of your sad psychopathology.'

He looked shocked and sat in silence for a long while. I watched him. He was staring at the books in my bookcase, avoiding eye contact. Eventually he started telling me about a Denzel Washington film he had seen at the weekend: 'Washington played an alcoholic. At the end of the film he was totally wasted. He had lost everything he ever cared about because of his addiction. His son said to him, "Dad, who are you?" The Washington character had been an addict for so long, pretending to be someone else for so long, even his son didn't know who he was. He was pathetic. I am pathetic.'

I was concerned that Lars was being so hard on himself, but I refrained from saying anything. He knew I cared, but I also thought maybe he needed to be hard on himself to survive this.

As Paula Hall points out in her book, the biggest problem for sex addicts, many of whom have experienced trauma in childhood, is that life is full of triggers for intense anxiety episodes. Lars and I had learned together to understand the causes of his addiction, but we agreed that he now needed a more specialised and cognitive approach to establish prevention strategies for managing and avoiding the many triggers in life. He began meditation classes, joined a sex addiction group and embarked on the 12-step programme. Just as for alcoholics and drug addicts, the road to recovery for sex addiction is long and hard.

8 On women's misogyny and self-hatred

Self-hatred and the angel in the house

Misogyny usually means men's hatred of women. But some women also experience intense feelings of hatred towards their own sex. Many women have been culturally conditioned not to resort to physical violence; nevertheless, there are many other ways for women to attack women such as emotional and verbal abuse, bullying and malicious gossip. But one of the most common manifestations of women's hatred of women is hatred turned inwards and directed against the self.

Self-attacks often take the form of self-harm. Cutting their arms or thighs with knives or razor blades is becoming increasingly common with some adolescent girls. Some women also punish their own bodies by starving themselves, or binge eating, which can also be physical manifestations of self-hatred. It used to be mainly older women who went through painful surgical procedures to supposedly make themselves younger, more beautiful and, so they believed, more lovable. But in this age of social media, young women are also paying plastic surgeons vast sums to give them a perfect face or a perfect body.

There are also women who are so convinced they are worthless they deliberately court dangerous situations. They drink or drug themselves into oblivion, they engage in relationships with abusive men, they work the streets as prostitutes, or they haunt the most dangerous areas of town late at night, tempting fate to punish them as proof of how bad and worthless they really are. In many women, I am tempted to say, some form of self-hatred has become almost normal.

Depression is one of the most pernicious and common forms of self-hatred. The writer, Virginia Woolf, was plagued by crippling episodes of depression and mania throughout her adult life which finally resulted in her suicide. In her essay 'Professions for Women' (1931), she wrote:

> every house had its Angel. And when I came to write I encountered her with the very first words. The shadow of her wings fell on my page; I heard the rustling of her skirts in the room. Directly, that is to say, I took my pen in my hand to review that novel by a famous man, she slipped behind me and whispered: 'My dear, you are a young woman. You are writing about a book that has been written by a man. Be sympathetic; be tender; flatter; deceive; use all the arts and wiles of our sex. Never let anybody guess that you have a mind of your own. Above all, be pure . . . .' I turned upon her and caught her by the throat. I did my best to kill her. My excuse, if I were to be had up in a court of law, would be that I acted in self-defence. Had I not killed her she would have killed me.

I can easily identify with Virginia Woolf's inner demons. I too have struggled with depressive episodes and an anxiety of authorship when struggling to write. Her rage with the greater power men have in culture and society is only part of the problem. She is also angry with the feminine wiles women are expected to employ to manipulate men to gain power through men as if by proxy. But isn't it interesting that when Virginia unleashes the full force of her rage, it is directed not against men but against the angel in the house? This angel is the female Virginia wants to kill, but who is she?

I think the angel represents another part of herself – the part that is self-destructive and smothering her sense of self-worth and her self-belief that she is good enough. I also think that at a more primitive level this hated 'angel in the house' embodies deeply ambivalent feelings towards the idealised, perfect mother. Virginia's mother died when she was 13. But Virginia said that it wasn't until she wrote her novel, *To the Lighthouse*, when she was 44, that she ceased to be obsessed with her mother:

> I no longer hear her voice; I do not see her. I suppose that I did for myself what psychoanalysts do for their clients. I expressed

> some very long felt and deeply felt emotion. And in expressing it I explained it and then laid it to rest.
>
> (1927)

I can imagine this 'deeply felt emotion' was a complex mixture of rage as well as love. The loss of your mother in your early teens is unbearably hard for anyone. But it must have been particularly hard for Virginia, whose mother was idealised as a paragon of virtue and feminine perfection. Virginia's mother was the impossible rival, the smothering angel in the house who had perniciously taken lodgings in a dark corner of Virginia's identity as a woman and a writer.

Although Virginia said through writing *To the Lighthouse* she had laid 'deeply felt emotion' to rest, it was just a temporary respite. She was sexually abused when she was six by her 20-year-old half-brother, Gerald. Years later she wrote that one of her strongest memories was a feeling of shame and guilt – a feeling which she described as 'the looking-glass of shame,' which 'has lasted all my life'. She briefly mentioned Gerald's abuse in a letter she wrote to a writer friend. In the letter, she congratulates her friend on the freedom with which she could write about masturbation and sex. This was something Virginia said she was unable to do herself. She wrote this letter a few weeks before her suicide in 1941 at the age of 59.

Virginia was also sexually abused by her other half-brother, George, when she was in her early teens. George had become her unofficial guardian shortly after her mother died. Virginia rarely mentioned the abuse. But after her suicide, a woman friend remembered a conversation she had with Virginia who told her that George used to often come to her bedroom at night to 'help her undress and paw her all over'.

It's not unusual for women who have been sexually abused in childhood to remain deeply angry with their mothers who failed to protect them. Virginia's mother's early death meant she was abandoned by her mother when she most needed her. We will never know the full extent of what George did to Virginia during those terrible years after her mother's death, but we do know that later she said it was George who 'sent me mad'. Episodes of depression and mania are common symptoms of post-traumatic stress disorder suffered by people who have been sexually abused in childhood. She was also deeply troubled by what she described as her 'inability to feel properly' and her sexual inhibition with her husband which blighted her marriage. She found some comfort in lesbian relationships, although she never left her husband. She remained emotionally dependent on him for most of her adult life.

Controlling mothers and sadomasochistic desires

As we have seen in earlier chapters, it's not unusual for women to feel a complicated mixture of love and mistrust or anger towards their mothers. I think this goes some way towards explaining why they nurture ambivalent feelings towards their own sex and themselves as women. But for a few women, their childhood relationship with their mother was so toxic, the result is an extreme self-hatred that poisons their capacity for intimacy and fulfilment in their sexual relationships with either sex in later life. Marie was one of these women.

Marie, in her late twenties, had grown up a Catholic in the South of Ireland. She said she needed therapy was because she was making such a mess of her life, particularly with men. She asked me if I had seen the film of *The Piano Teacher*. She looked disappointed when I shook my head. 'The film is about me,' she said, with great conviction. 'I mean it's not really about me. But I thought if you had seen the film it might help you to understand me.' I was intrigued, of course, and the following weekend I downloaded the DVD. The story of *The Piano Teacher* turned out to be one of the most disturbing films about a woman's sexuality I have ever seen.

I will tell you about *The Piano Teacher* before talking about Marie's story. The film is adapted from a novel by the Austrian author Elfriede Jelinek who won the Nobel Prize for Literature in 2004. Jelinek confessed that aspects of the novel contain autobiographical elements. She was probably referring to the way her heroine, Erika, was forced by her ambitious, overbearing mother to submit to a gruelling regime of training as a concert pianist. The story explores the devastating impact a mother's determination to control every aspect of her daughter's life has on her daughter's sexuality.

Erika, in her late thirties, teaches piano at the Vienna Conservatoire. As a teacher she is a bullying disciplinarian who terrifies her students. Erika has no friends and lives in a claustrophobic apartment with her mother – her father was committed to a mental institution soon after Erika was born. Over the years the mother-daughter relationship has become enmeshed like a dysfunctional married couple; they are tied to each other by mutual dependency and mutual antagonism and the tension between them is unbearable. Erika has never had a life of her own and she has never had any privacy, not even the privacy to masturbate. She has a small sitting room of her own, but the room doesn't have a lock, and for her entire life she has shared a bedroom with her mother, sleeping on her father's side of the double bed. As Jelinek put it, 'Erika has no chance to caress herself. Her mother sleeps next to her and guards Erika's hands. These hands are supposed to practice, not scoot under the blanket like ants and scurry over to the jam jar.' Similarly, she has never been allowed boyfriends. 'Mother threatens to kill the child if she ever so much as sees her with a man. Mother keeps her eyes peeled, she checks, hunts, calculates, concludes, punishes.' Erika's only relief from her mother's strict regime is self-harm; she shuts herself in the bathroom whilst her mother is cooking and cuts her thighs with a razor blade.

The damage done to Erika's sexuality is extreme. She's gained her sexual education from hardcore movies she views in the porn shops. She has also become a voyeur, visiting dangerous districts of Vienna at night where she lurks in the shadows spying on prostitutes having sex with their johns.

Erika nurtures sadistic and masochistic fantasies and is quite capable of launching her own sadistic attacks. Now in her late thirties, she is plagued by thoughts of her lost youth and her aging body and is consumed by jealousy when she sees Walter, one of her handsome young students at the Conservatoire, eyeing a pretty, young female pianist. She takes her revenge on the girl by breaking a glass and placing the shards into the girl's coat pocket – the girl's hand is so badly cut, her chances of performing are ruined.

Walter is something of a Don Juan in the student world and he is determined to add his teacher to his sexual conquests. He visits Erika at her apartment, much to her mother's fury. They manage to shut mother out of Erika's room and Walter tries to seduce her. But instead of responding as he expects, Erika shows him the contents of an old shoebox she keeps hidden that contains ropes, handcuffs, chains, gags. She insists he reads a letter she has written listing her instructions for the things he must do to her if they are to have sex. He must tie her up, gag her, slap and beat her, and he must threaten her loudly if she refuses. Walter is repulsed by her request and walks out of the apartment in disgust. He is also puzzled. 'Did he get it right? By becoming her master, he can never become her master? So long as she dictates what he should do to her, some final remnant of Erika will remain unfathomable.'

The humiliation and shame Erika feels having revealed her secret masochistic desires, only to be rejected, is unbearable. She goes to the bedroom where her mother furiously chastises her for having a man in the apartment. Erika's response is extraordinary and deeply disturbing; she climbs on top of her mother who is already in bed and attempts to have sex with her: 'It's like a lover's struggle, and the goal isn't orgasm, but Mother per se . . . Erika sucks and gnaws on this big body as if she wanted to crawl back into it and hide inside it.' Her mother's reaction is disgust; she forces her daughter off her and accuses her of being crazy.

What was Erika doing, trying to have sex with her mother? Was she manifesting her craving for the love her mother has never been able to give her? Or was this attempt at sex with her mother a furious attack; her only way of communicating that her sexual needs were overwhelming her, and she can't see any way that they can ever be fulfilled by anyone except her mother? Her attempt at sex with her mother reveals both a desperate need for her mother's love and at the same time a hate-fuelled attack on her mother who has deprived her of her freedom and condemned her to a life of sexual repression. Erika's sexual craving to be literally bound, gagged and beaten is the psychological price she is paying for having lived her entire life as if she has been bound, gagged and beaten, cut off as she has been from a normal childhood and normal sexual development. For Erika, the only intimacy she has ever known has been with her mother and that has been a constant power struggle between control and subjugation, domination and submission.

Erika may appear 'crazy', as her mother said, but it is her mother who has made her what she is. But as Jelinek makes clear in the novel, this toxic mother-daughter relationship does not exist in a vacuum. The context of these women's lives – the male-dominated hierarchical world of the Conservatoire and the grimy, sadistic and violent underworld of the sex industry – is exploitative of women and deeply misogynist. The manifestations in society of this hatred of women and the determination to dominate and control women, is exemplified, towards the end of the story, by Erika's student, Walter. He returns to her apartment and brutally rapes her, insisting that he is merely giving her what she asked for. Erika is undoubtedly a seriously disturbed woman who has both masochistic and sadistic sexual fantasies, but nurturing a confused fantasy of being tied up, gagged and dominated is quite a different thing from wanting to be raped. For Erika, as it would be for any other woman, the reality of rape is traumatic and terrifying.

What compelled Marie to pick up men who disgusted her?

Marie looked a little like a younger version of Isabelle Huppert, who played Erika in the film. On the surface, her appearance exuded a healthy air of normality: reddish blond curls, green eyes, freckles, smart, well cared-for clothes, sensible shoes. But the physical appearance of both Marie, and of Erika, was deceptive. It wasn't their physical resemblance that Marie was referring to when she asked if I had seen the film; the similarities went deeper.

Early in her therapy, Marie told me she had seen a therapist once before, for just a few sessions. She hinted that something had once happened to her sexually, but she couldn't tell me what it was. She said she had made the mistake of telling this other therapist. He had judged her and blamed her for what had happened. She was afraid to tell me because I would do the same. I wondered if this ex-therapist really had judged her, or if Marie had projected her own harsh inner judge onto the therapist. Whatever, I knew I would have to be patient and wait until Marie trusted me enough to tell me what she had done that was so bad.

Marie often laughed cheerfully when she walked into my room for her therapy session, as if she didn't have a care in the world. But as I soon learnt, her carefree ripples of laughter were also a protective shield; her defence against anyone, including me, getting too close. She used her flirtatiousness and seductive charm in a similar way. I often felt the need to resist her drawing me in and manipulating me. She was amused when I told her this, but at the same time I think she was relieved that I wasn't falling for her usual games. She was testing me. Her distress, when she finally revealed the full extent of her vulnerability, was so great she needed to trust that I was strong enough to cope with who she really was.

Marie said that she had never had a good sexual relationship or any kind of lasting real relationship with a man. However, she insisted that all she wanted was a nice, normal man, a secure home and children. But if a man she really liked showed any interest in her, she couldn't bear it. She would drink too much, behave badly and be nasty to him to drive him away. The only way she could have sex, or even let a man kiss her, was if she was drunk. She frequently fell into self-destructive moods when she didn't care if she lived or died. She loitered around seedy low-life bars late at night, drank too much and got picked up by men who disgusted her. Something compelled her to seek out sex with these kinds of men. Afterwards she felt worthless and filled with self-disgust. She knew she had been lucky so far; it was only a matter of time before one of these men seriously hurt her.

Marie said she enjoyed pretending to be a femme fatale; she liked feeling powerful and seductive. But she admitted that it was also a way of covering up her feelings of intense vulnerability. For her, the intimacy of a loving sexual relationships was almost unbearable. The question was why, as this was the thing she said she most wanted.

Marie said she was the black sheep in her family. She was also convinced that she had ruined her mother's life. If her mother hadn't got pregnant in her teens, she would never have married Marie's father who, according to her mother and grandmother, was a low-life drunk. Her mother left him when Marie was two years old. She later remarried and had two more children. Her stepfather was only interested in his own children. Marie felt like the unwanted, unloved outsider in her stepfamily. Her mother blamed Marie for everything that was wrong in her life – her depressions, her lack of professional achievements, her conviction that she was growing old before her time. She even blamed Marie for looking like her father: the sight of Marie was a constant reminder of the wicked man who had ruined her. Marie used to wonder if her father really was as wicked as her mother and grandmother claimed. But she also felt rejected by her father and very angry with him. If he cared about her, he would have come to find her and rescue her from her mother. But he never came.

When Marie was 13, her mother declared that her behaviour had become so bad she was out of control and a bad influence on her half-siblings. They would all be better off without her. Marie was sent to live with her grandmother in another town. She was told that now her grandmother was old she needed Marie to do the housework and the shopping. Also, her grandmother was a strict disciplinarian who wouldn't put up with any bad behaviour: 'I was expected to go to school and to be her unpaid servant at her beck and call the rest of the time.'

Marie was forced to leave her old school and her friends behind, and despite everything, she loved her mother and her half-siblings. Her grandmother's flat was much too small for the two of them. She had to share her grandmother's double bed which she hated. Sharing a bed with an old lady had disgusted her. She comforted herself in bed at night by telling herself that when she grew up, she would become a nun: 'I had this fantasy of me turning up at home one day in my nun's habit. I would look at the surprise on their faces and give them a beneficent smile. That would prove to my mother and grandmother that they were wrong about me, I really was good. But I knew, even then, this wasn't true. I was bad, like they said. That was why my mother sent me away.'

'So, you had behaved badly,' I said. 'Lots of children do when they are unhappy. But that doesn't make you intrinsically bad. I think you were the scapegoat.'

Marie looked alert: 'I liked the story of the scapegoat at school. The poor old goat, loaded up with the sins of the Israelites and driven out into the desert.'

'Exactly, they projected their sins, or bad feelings, onto the goat and drove it away to make them feel better. I think this is what your mother was doing, projecting all her bad feelings about herself onto you. You weren't bad, any more than that poor scapegoat was bad.'

'Yes, it's nice that you think that. But I know I am bad.' Marie smiled sweetly.

There was something about Marie's false sweet smile that always alerted me to when she was hiding something. 'Marie, don't you think it will soon be time to tell me whatever it was you told your previous therapist that you think was so bad?'

'I will think about it,' she tossed out, casually, as she walked out of the door.

The next week she arrived for her session in a highly anxious state. She sat in silence for a while staring at me, as if she was thinking about whether to trust me or not. Finally, she said had decided to risk it. She told me about a night when she was 14. She had a furious row with her grandmother and walked out. She had already begun hanging out in seedy bars pretending to be older than she was. That night she went to a bar, got drunk and went to an area of town near the station where prostitutes touted for business. She was picked up in a car by a man who thought she was a prostitute and paid her for sex.

'That was how I lost my virginity.' She sobbed. 'This is proof of how worthless I really am. A good man would never love me if he knew the truth about my past.'

'I don't think it proves anything,' I said. 'Marie, you were a lonely, unhappy, child who felt unwanted and unloved. The man in the car who picked you up that night and raped you is to blame, not you.'

'It wasn't rape,' she managed to say. 'I took the money. I consented, I was drunk, but I knew what I was doing. It was my fault.'

'You were fourteen. You were a child,' I said, 'Don't you think it's time for you to stop blaming yourself?' I watched as she grabbed a handful of tissues to wipe her nose. She looked like a 14-year-old child.

Marie knew she needed therapy. She knew she was on a crash course to self-annihilation, and she desperately needed help. But getting her to let go of her belief that she was bad was an uphill struggle.

Unlike Erika, Marie was likeable, kind, empathetic and she had close friends who cared about her. I think she chose *The Piano Teacher* as a way of telling me about herself because she needed me to see beyond her false self. She knew, if the therapy was to do any good, we would need to grapple with the dark, destructive and self-destructive recesses of her character. Like Erika, Marie liked to despise normal people. She looked down on them leading their boring, narrow little lives, just as she looked down on her stepfamily. She needed to despise them because this was her defence against her conviction that they despised her. Also, Marie, like Erika, was compulsively drawn to the sexual underworld. When she was drunk and flirting with the men she despised in seedy all-night bars, she may have hated herself but at the same time she knew these men were beneath her, she was better than them. She enjoyed getting high on her seductive, sexual power over them. She was excited by the danger; there was a kind of heady liberation, throwing caution to the wind, believing that it didn't matter what happened to her because nobody really cared about her and she didn't care either. She believed this was her truth; she was bravely staring the truth in the eye.

She also identified with Erika's conflicted, ambivalent feelings towards her mother. Somewhere, deep inside her, Marie longed for a mother's unconditional love. Like Erika, she longed to crawl back into her mother's big body and 'hide away inside it'. But, like Erika, her love for her mother was inextricably mixed up with rage. Rage, hatred and self-hatred were safe feelings, they were her only defence against the extreme vulnerability she felt in all intimate relationships. This was why it was so hard for her to allow a man, or woman, to get too close to her, including me.

After about a year of therapy Marie told me that she had decided to go and live in another part of the country with a new boyfriend. I was concerned, I knew she was bound to have another crisis and would need more help. I wished her well and gave her the name of a therapist I knew who lived in the city she was moving to.

A few years later I sent her this piece I had written about our work together. She replied with a long email telling me about the messy ending of her relationship with her boyfriend ten months earlier. But she had taken up my suggestion to continue therapy: 'I have been seeing [the therapist] since June last year – once a week and if there is a crisis sometimes twice a week. From my perspective the first six months is just a waste of time, talking about things that aren't really important, building trust, pretending, manipulating etc., but even though things are still tough I can now feel that a shift has happened . . . but this is only the beginning. . . . the very beginning, but I refuse to give up and ruin my life, and I am not my mother or grandmother. . . . I will have a life worth living, promise!!!!

Cherry it's absolutely fine, you have got my permission to use the work that we have done together as a part of your book.'

At the end of her email she had added this PS: 'PS sometimes I wish my ex-boyfriend would become really ill, so I could look after him like the French girl in *Bitter Moon* looked after her lover who really hurt her (movie by Roman Polanski), but this is only a fantasy, and let's leave it like that. :-)'

She was hooking me into another film I hadn't seen. I googled *Bitter Moon* and discovered the film was about extreme sado-masochism. The protagonist was a woman who my favourite film reviewer, Roger Ebert, described as 'a voracious seductress with black widow tendencies whose amusement is to blind men in the headlights of her sexuality.' As I read about the film, I could almost hear Marie's playful laughter.

On domination, submission and sadomasochism

Vivienne came to see me to tell me she was fine about me telling her story. But she had a few concerns. It was important to her that people understood that BDSM had liberated her sexually – it was the bit of her relationship that had worked. It was also important to her that I explained BDSM properly. She didn't like the way BDSM had been misrepresented in *Fifty Shades of Grey*, which then was a recent bestseller. I shall return to Vivienne's story later. But first, I need to do my best to fulfil Vivienne's wishes and explain BDSM.

BDSM, or bondage, discipline and sadomasochism, involves one partner playing the role of the dominant, master or madam, whilst the other partner takes the role of the submissive, dog, bitch or slave. The methods of control typically include a variety of shackles: handcuffs, dog collars, ropes, chains, gags, blindfolds and implements for inflicting punishment and pain such as belts and whips. Dressing up and ritual are an important part of the practice.

A quick look at BDSM on Wikipedia shows that there is nothing new about the practice. Early frescoes have been found that depict whipping and flagellation as forms of sexual arousal. Some ancient texts describe sexual rituals that are 'imbued with pain and ecstasy bringing about initiation and journeys of altered states of consciousness; punishment, moaning, ecstasy, lament and song, participants exhausting themselves in weeping and grief'. The *Kama Sutra* refers to 'four kinds of hitting during love making' and mentions the importance of safety rules when practicing sadomasochistic sex: 'as only some women consider such practices joyful or playful'.

The assumption in the *Kama Sutra* appears to be that it is women who are the submissives. But whilst research has shown that more women than men are attracted to the submissive role, the BDSM literature points out that the roles are not gender specific. It's also important to make a distinction between BDSM sexual practices and the kind of misogynistic male violence and sexual abuse of women that takes place in the general population.

Unlike most sexual violence, BDSM rituals begin with a negotiation between consenting adults to establish the rules and boundaries of the session. Safe words are established – usually colours: red for 'stop', and yellow or amber for 'slow down' or 'pause'. 'Yes' and 'no' are ruled out as safe words as they are often uttered spontaneously during sex. Empathy for your sexual partner is also important, to enable you to remain aware of your partner's psychological triggers so that emotional overload, breakdowns and actual physical harm can be avoided.

Freud was interested in sadomasochism. He begins his essay 'The Sexual Aberrations' (1905b), by pointing out that sadomasochistic desires are on the spectrum of normal sexual behaviour which necessarily contains elements of both aggressiveness and submissiveness. But in more extreme cases, sadism is a violent or aggressive attitude towards your sexual partner where 'satisfaction is entirely conditional on their humiliation and maltreatment.' Masochism can also be any passive attitude towards sexual life and the sexual object, but in extreme cases it is when satisfaction can only be achieved through 'suffering physical or mental pain at the hands of the sexual object.'

For Freud, this raised a perplexing question: when can sexual inclinations, even if they are unusual, be termed a pathology or a perversion? He resolved this quandary, in his own mind at least, by making a distinction between the so-called normal, if wide-ranging, variations in sexual inclinations, and a specific sexual behaviour at the further end of the spectrum which, as he put it, 'ousts completely' all variations and takes on the characteristics of 'exclusiveness and fixation'. This, he thought, could be 'justified . . . as a pathological symptom.'

A 2013 psychological study (which took the form of an Internet questionnaire) found that, when compared to a control group, 'BDSM practitioners were less neurotic, more extroverted, more open to new experiences, more conscientious, less rejection sensitive, had a higher subjective well-being, yet were less agreeable than vanillas' (vanillas are people who confine themselves to 'normal' sexual practices). It's impossible to know what to make of this without knowing what the researchers meant by terms such as 'less neurotic' and 'less agreeable'. However, it could indicate that participants in the BDSM subculture have found a sexual outlet for their particular 'neuroses,' which includes the healthy practice of talking to each other about their sexual preferences and emotional hang-ups, whilst the 'vanillas' in the control group reflected the kind of 'normal neuroses' experienced by the majority of sexually confused, repressed people in the general population when it comes to managing their sexual lives. On the other hand, it could simply reflect the fact that it's not unusual for people who identify with a subgroup, whatever that subgroup's particular sexual preference, to feel beleaguered, marginalised and misunderstood by the rest of society. Given the long history of persecution suffered by sexually marginalised subgroups, they are, understandably, keen for their preferences to be accepted and not labelled as neurotic or pathological. The study concluded that 'BDSM may be thought of as recreational leisure, rather than the expression of psychopathological processes.'

It seems to me that whether a sexual practice is abnormal or pathological isn't really an issue, so long as it is practiced without coercion between mutually consenting adults who are fully informed and know what they are doing. The problems arise if the sexual practice is causing psychological or physical harm or distress to the practitioners that is beyond the intended sexual stimulation. However, like all the sexual relationships I have talked about so far in this book, I think it is likely that the roots of the BDSM practitioners' sexual preferences lie in their childhood attachments and early sexual development. I don't see any reason why people in the BDSM community should be any different from the rest of the population in this regard.

How Vivienne found herself through bondage

Vivienne, in her late thirties, was bright, attractive, self-assured and appeared to be very much in control of her life. She and a friend had set up a successful business specialising in vintage clothes and historical costumes. She was also bringing up her 12-year-old daughter, Sally, on her own. She said she was struggling with anxiety and depression. She had had individual therapy in the past and dealt with her childhood issues, and she really didn't want to go back over the childhood stuff again. A friend had recommended group therapy. Did I think group therapy might help her? And did I have a space for her in my therapy group?

A man in my weekly long-term group had recently left the group. This meant I did have a space for one new person. But I needed to get to know Vivienne before I could say whether I thought a therapy group might be right for her. I explained that feelings connected to childhood experiences inevitably come up in groups. An important part of the work of a group is to learn to recognise these feelings and to use the group to explore how they might be affecting our current relationships, that is relationships formed within the group as well as those outside the group with partners, family, friends, work colleagues and so forth. I suggested we start with some individual sessions and then we decide about the group.

The following week it was as if a different woman walked into my consulting room. Vivienne collapsed into tears almost immediately. She said she was desperate, she felt as if she was falling apart. Her boyfriend, Tom, had ended their relationship the previous day. The thought of losing him was unbearable: 'I asked him if we could plan for a short holiday, to fit in with my daughter's half term. All I wanted was to book a hotel, to give my daughter a holiday to look forward to. He sent me a text telling me it was demands like this that made him realise our relationship was never going to work. And he just ended it.' She dissolved into tears again. 'That's the problem. If I ask Tom for anything, he accuses me of making demands. He refuses to even talk about our relationship or to make plans. He says I am making demands, which he hates. He won't even make plans for next week. I never know when we will see each other again. If I press him too much he closes up completely, and then he goes back to his place and won't answer the phone or to see me until he's ready.'

'He sounds like a difficult man to have a relationship with,' I said, cautiously.

'I don't know, maybe I'm the one who is difficult. I'm so confused. He's completely changed my life. It's because of him I have come alive. Before I met Tom, I never liked sex, but sex with him is amazing. I discovered I had a body and a whole range of feelings I didn't know existed. I can't stand the thought of losing him.'

I could feel myself beginning to dislike Tom. But it was good to know he was a great lover. So not all bad, I told myself as I watched Vivienne grabbing more tissues from the box. I reminded myself that it was early days and I didn't know Tom's side of the story.

'I've tried not to ask him for anything, but he still thinks I'm trying to control him,' Vivienne continued. 'I know he's got issues to do with his controlling mother. His father died in a road accident when Tom was five and his mother wouldn't let him out of her sight from then on, in case something happened to him too. I've got control issues with my mother too. I've suggested couple therapy, but he refuses. He says I'm the one who should be in therapy.'

Control, or lack of control, had been a huge issue for Vivienne when she was growing up. Her mother had controlled her every move with relentless verbal attacks and regular beatings. Her older sister, her mother's favourite, also bullied her. Their father, Vivienne said, was a weak, pathetic man who did nothing to rescue Vivienne from his wife and older daughter's abuse. The only way Vivienne could defend herself in her family was to be completely obedient, never to get in the way or annoy her mother, and not to speak unless spoken to. Her survival strategy was to make herself invisible in the hope that her mother wouldn't notice her because to be noticed meant she was in danger of being attacked. All the while, she secretly fantasised about escaping. She was 14 when she ran away from home. She hid in a barn for two days until the police found her and took her home. As soon as she was old enough to leave school, she packed her bags and left home for good. Since then she had contacted her family only very occasionally to let them know where she was living. Her daughter, Sally, had never met her grandparents.

After a few sessions we returned to the subject of the group. Given the strong theme of scapegoating and rejection in her family story, I thought powerful feelings were bound to come up for her in the therapy group which can feel a little like another family. There would probably be times when she would want run from the group, just as she had wanted to escape from her family. It would be important for her not to keep these feelings to herself but to work through them in the group. Was she still sure she wanted to join the group? She nodded. She recognised that the group was an opportunity for her to grow. She had made up her mind.

Just before the end of her final individual session – she was due to join the group the following week – she told me she had written Tom a letter. She was still distressed that she hadn't heard from him and she wanted him to know how she felt. She said it was a short letter, just a description of her picture of their relationship that she wanted him to have. In the picture Tom, a skilled craftsman, was sitting at his work bench getting on with whatever piece he was carving. Vivienne was in a dark corner of his workroom wearing a long white dress. She was tied up and gagged, watching him silently. I assumed this disturbing image of herself was intended as a metaphor, a way of telling Tom how she felt in their relationship. But it was the end of her session, there wasn't time to talk about what the image meant to her. I would have to wait until she was ready to bring it up in the group.

Vivienne and Tom got back together soon after she joined the group. But it was far from plain sailing. Also, I noticed a pattern soon develop in the group as Vivienne oscillated between two positions. In some sessions she was expressive, open, vulnerable, as she shared the highs and the lows of her on-off relationship with Tom. In these sessions she was vocal and articulate; she empathised with other group members and seemed interested in what they had to say. But in other sessions she would remain almost totally silent for the whole group with a frozen, mask-like expression on her face. These silences made some members of the group nervous. Long silences can serve as a vacuum for projections. Two women in the group said they found her silence frightening; they were convinced that she was angry with them. A man in the group said he didn't want to be like her apathetic father – he wanted to connect with her, but he didn't know how to if she wouldn't tell him what she was feeling. Occasionally I would ask her if she was alright. I wanted to help her to come out of her shell. Sometimes this worked, and she would begin to join in and talk about the themes that had come up that resonated with her. Just because she had been silent, that didn't mean she hadn't been listening. On these occasions I could almost hear the group breathe a sigh of relief; she was back. But on other occasions she would say she was fine, but the look in her eyes when I spoke to her directly was startled and bewildered, like a frightened rabbit caught in the headlights – like the frightened child she had once been in her childhood family when her mother attacked her.

One day when she was in a good mood, she suddenly decided to tell the group how she had met Tom: 'It was at a fetish party. That's dressing up and sex games,' she added for the benefit of a group member who didn't know what a fetish party was. 'It had been just a fun night out with a girlfriend. Then I met Tom and he introduced me to BDSM. He explained about the rules and the safe words. This made me feel safe, I knew that he wouldn't really hurt me. The first time he tied me up was frightening but soon I discovered feelings I had never experienced before. I discovered I liked sex. I could feel his kindness and his concern for my feelings. It was the first time I have ever trusted a man completely. Once I got really carried away; I couldn't stop weeping. I think these feelings came from deep down and way back in my childhood. Tom saw what was going on and realised that I had forgotten to use the safe word. He stopped the session and comforted me and told me he loved me. After that everything was fine.'

The group were completely silent as they listened to Vivienne's revelation. One woman said she couldn't imagine allowing anyone to tie her up; she would be far too scared. But she liked hearing Vivienne talking so confidently about sex. Instead of the judgement Vivienne had expected, the group were inspired to talk about the many conflicts, dilemmas and secret desires they were struggling with in their own sex lives. Their discussion ranged from pornography and shameful sexual fantasies to feelings of deep sadness when sex has died in a long-term relationship.

Over the following months the group continued to try to understand Vivienne and Tom's relationship. They thought it was great that Vivienne felt sexually liberated by BDSM, but how did that fit with the rest of Vivienne's relationship with Tom? We had heard a lot about Tom's withholding behaviour since Vivienne joined the group, and we had all witnessed Vivienne's distress on the occasions when Tom ended their relationship. Was BDSM Tom's way to avoid commitment? Was 'normal' intimacy unbearable for Tom? Maybe it was for Vivienne too? Vivienne said she had asked Tom for more intimacy when they had sex, but as usual he had taken her request as a sign that their relationship wasn't working. Now they were seeing each other again, she was trying to learn to accept him as he was, not to ask for anything, not to have needs of her own. The group found it difficult to accept that Vivienne thought the solution was to deny that she had needs of her own. It seemed that Tom was in control of the entire relationship; he not only bound and gagged her sexually, he was also tying her up and gagging her emotionally. Life with Tom may have been sexually liberating, but the rest of their relationship was beginning to seem like emotional torture.

One-day Vivienne came to the group in great distress. She said that Tom had introduced a new element into their sexual relationship without negotiating with her first. He had invited another woman, a stranger, to watch. She hated this woman being there; she felt horribly vulnerable but unable to do anything about it because she was tied up and gagged. What made the situation worse for her was that afterwards when she tried to talk to Tom about it, he refused to discuss it. She was very distressed by this new development; he had broken the rules that made her feel safe. She also confessed that sometimes she was afraid she was becoming addicted. Now she had discovered that she liked sex when she's tied up, she liked being completely passive, being given orders, and having things done to her, she liked it when nothing was expected of her – she was afraid that she couldn't live without it.

Vivienne was beginning to realise that she was caught in a contradiction between the part of her that pined for loving intimacy and the part of her that turned her back on intimacy because she didn't like the feeling of anyone getting too close to her. Apart from her relationship with her daughter, who made her feel warm and safe, this conflict was present in all her relationships, including her relationship with the group. This also, at least partly explained why sometimes she would come to the group and be warm and responsive to the group, whilst on other occasions she would retreat into her silent shell. She said she had given up wanting her mother's love a long time ago. But she admitted there may be a psychological similarity between her relationship with Tom and how she used to be as a child, when she used to sit very still and be too afraid to speak because she was terrified of her mother's sudden violent attacks. Tom was never violently attacking like her mother, but he controlled her by withholding his affection and refusing to meet any of her needs, except when they were having sex and he was in control in his role as the dominant. During her time in the group she came to understand that her submissive role in their sex ritual, when she was bound, gagged and punished, was a kind of re-enactment from her childhood. The difference was that the sexual excitement aroused by the ritual gave her an overwhelming feeling of relief. Ironically, given that she was tied up, she felt freed from something. She wondered if she was freed from guilt. When she was being punished, she was freed from a nagging feeling that she must have been guilty of something bad which was why her mother hated her. She may also have been freed from her own vengeful impulses rooted in her rage with her mother for hurting her. And she was freed from her deep longing for her mother's love, a love that had always been withheld from her – the sexual ritual released her from that longing because, whatever Tom withheld from her in the rest of their relationship, during the ritual she felt entirely satisfied and completely loved.

Some people in the group wondered if an equivalent re-enactment was happening for Tom. The part of the dominant meant he was completely in control within the limits provided by the rules and boundaries. This enabled him to feel safe enough to express his sadistic impulses knowing he wouldn't really hurt her, as well as his feelings of love and affection. The sexual ritual freed him from the danger of real intimacy. But why was Tom afraid of intimacy? Had his mother held him too close after his father's death? Did he experience intimacy as suffocating? Was this why the problems in the relationship began when the sexual rituals were over. Vivienne wanted Tom's reassurance that he loved her. But this caused Tom to withdraw from her. Withholding affection and resisting Vivienne's requests for intimacy, which he experienced as demands, was his way of defending himself.

Whatever, Tom wasn't in the group and Vivienne was. And we were concerned for her. Tom's withholding behaviour, and his constant threats to abandon her and repeated actual abandonments, were unbearable, not least because they tapped into her unconscious childhood fears that her mother hated her and might one day abandon her. But whatever the group's concerns, both Tom and Vivienne appeared to be stuck in this vicious cycle with the BDSM sexual rituals their only alleviation from their psychological pain.

Until one day when Vivienne came to the group with an image she recalled from the previous night's dream. The image was a child's doll that was tied up and gagged. She said she knew, as soon as she woke up, that the doll was both herself as a child and herself as Tom's plaything. A few weeks after the dream, she and Tom went to a 'swinging party' (where couples swap sexual partners). Now she was even more confused, because she had enjoyed 'vanilla' sex with a man she met at the party who was kind and attentive to her needs. As a result, she was no longer sure what she felt about Tom.

I thought this could be a sign that Vivienne was changing. I didn't want to risk voicing this thought in the group; change is a delicate thing and I didn't want to stop it in its tracks. But it was soon after this event that Vivienne decided it was time for her to leave the group. She had been in the group for 18 months. She had gained a lot from the group, but she had gone as far as she wanted to go. The group said they felt sad she was leaving. They wanted her to stay for longer. But this expression of affection for her made Vivienne uncomfortable. 'I hate it when people are being nice to me,' she said. 'Being nice gives me a feeling of disgust, like a physical revulsion. I don't trust it.'

The group were confused and hurt by her reaction. It felt as if she was trying to undo all the good work we had done together. It also confirmed my feeling that Vivienne was leaving the group too soon. I thought she was leaving because she was afraid of becoming attached to the group. She was afraid of losing the distance she felt she needed to feel safe. But Vivienne was adamant that it was time for her to leave and I believed her when she said she had gained a lot from the group. She had gone as far as she could go for the time being. Sometimes it is only over time that we know if, and how, therapy has changed us.

When Vivienne came to see me a few years later, she told me she had changed. Her relationship with Tom had ended. She was now in a relationship with a loving man who was fine with dressing up and playing sex games, but they weren't allowing it to become 'a fixation'. They also enjoyed 'vanilla sex'.

I think Vivienne's story tells us that some people, men and women, find themselves sexually liberated by the strict rituals of BDSM. The fact that the practice includes couples talking to each other about sexual preferences, as well as stressing the importance of mutually agreed rules and empathy for each other's feelings, is also an important lesson that many 'vanillas' could benefit from.

In 2013 Amy Bonomi published a detailed analysis of *Fifty Shades of Grey*. She was careful to make a distinction between the ritualised practice of BDSM and the manipulative ploys of Grey, the novel's male protagonist, which are typical of abusive men: stalking, coercion, intimidation, humiliation, physical threats and actual physical violence. She pointed out that 'within the context of consensual BDSM relationships, substance abuse [alcohol] negates consent, negotiation and contracts are taken seriously, and boundaries are respected.' She also discusses the occasions in the novel when the heroine, Anastasia, who was still a virgin when Grey introduced her to BDSM, expressed her extreme confusion and fear in response to Grey's behaviour towards her. For instance, when Anastasia complained of feeling demeaned, debased and abused, Grey criticised her for not behaving like a proper submissive who would embrace these feelings and deal with them, for him. In other words, he made her feel there was something wrong with her, she was inadequate for not fulfilling his wishes. This is typical 'gaslighting' behaviour (i.e. manipulating your partner in such a way that it causes them to believe there is something very wrong with them and ultimately to lose their trust in their own sense of reality). Sadly, there will always be some people who are narcissistic, lack empathy or respect for their partners, and behave abusively, irrespective of whether their sexual preference is BDSM or 'vanilla'.

9 On passion, envy, rage and hate

What Melanie Klein told us about love and hate

> Love and hate are struggling together in the baby's mind; and this struggle to a certain extent persists throughout life and is liable to become a source of danger in human relationships.
>
> —Melanie Klein (1937)

Some men hate the women they love so much that they viciously attack them. Domestic violence statistics tell us that 31 percent of women – that's almost one in three – have been assaulted by their partners or ex-partners. Women are not always the innocent victims: they can be nasty, cruel, sadistic, vengeful, fly into hate-filled rages and violently abuse their partners. Domestic abuse also takes place in gay relationships. In Chapter 5, Heather talked about the abuse she had suffered in her lesbian relationships. But it's rare for women to murder their partners or ex-partners, whereas on average two women a week are murdered by their partner or ex-partner. The stark statistic remains: heterosexual men are more likely to kill their female partners; women who murder their partners are more likely to do so in self-defence. Is this because more women have been culturally conditioned not to express their hatred with extreme violence? Or could it be that when it comes to extreme violent hatred in sexual relationships, men and women behave differently?

Of all psychoanalytic theories, I think Melanie Klein's work comes closest to revealing the primitive roots of this toxic combination of love and hate, as well as a gamut of closely related emotions: extreme rage, the urge to destroy the person we love, the fear of destroying them, envy, rivalry, jealousy, guilt, the fear of being abandoned by the person we love, and the powerful need, after the rage has wreaked havoc, to make everything alright again.

Klein based her analytic theory mainly on her work with infants and young children. Research into these crucial early years, carried out by the Anna Freud Centre and proponents of attachment theory, has come a long way since Klein. Nevertheless Klein, like Freud, leaves us with a legacy of brilliant, imaginative and thought-provoking insights that, like great works of art, probe beyond the reach of evidence-based research into the heart of the matter.

When I was training as a psychotherapist, of all the various psychoanalytic theories I studied, I found Klein's writing the most difficult to grasp. It was worth the struggle: I have frequently found myself thinking about her ideas when trying to understand the deeper and darker recesses of love and hate. But how to make her ideas accessible for readers without getting lost in psychoanalytic abstractions? I had been worrying about this problem for some time when *The Weeping Woman* (1937), Picasso's cubist portrait, came into my mind and I had an idea. If Melanie Klein had been an artist, surely, she would never have painted soft focus, pastel pink, naturalistic mothers and babies. She would have painted extraordinary, disturbing and highly dramatic images like Picasso. Could I try describing Klein's theories visually as if they were an imaginary exhibition of Picasso prints – variations on the theme of mother and child?

My imaginary Melanie Klein exhibition

In the first room of the exhibition, at first glance the pictures appear to consist of bewildering distortions of breasts and nipples and, in amongst these bits of mother, the eyes and hands of a greedy baby determined to get what it wants. But as we look at the detail, we see that in the first picture the baby's hands are grabbing at the breasts as if they are kneading them like baker's dough, and the baby's mouth is sucking her nipples, its eyes semi-closed in blissful contentment – mother is good and loving, baby is satisfied, and all is well in baby's world. But not for long. In the next picture there's something wrong: the baby can't get satisfaction. Its face has become distorted by frustration, greed and rage. The baby's eyes are livid green: it's consumed by envy for what it wants that it cannot have. It attacks and tears furiously at the breasts as if it is intent on destruction.

The baby's envious attack leads us to the theme of the next set of pictures: paranoia! The pictures are violent and chaotic depicting how the baby's rage-fuelled attacks are being projected into bits of breasts. In *Love, Guilt and Reparation* (1937) Klein tells us that:

> [the baby's] hatred and aggressive feelings are aroused, and he becomes dominated by the impulse to destroy the very person [mother] who is the object of all his desires and who in his mind is linked to everything he experiences, good and bad alike.

The result of all this hatred and rage is that the baby experiences an acute paranoid anxiety – it becomes afraid that the object of its attack [its mother] may become monstrous, take her revenge and attack back! Klein gives us this brilliant insight into the workings of paranoia: 'the object that arouses guilt turns into a persecutor'.

The tone of the next set of pictures is quite different; each image is split into two very different parts. In one half we see the perfect, good, loving mother with her satisfied infant. In the other half we see the monstrous, attacking bad mother with her fearful, hate-filled infant. What these pictures tell us is that the infant has become so threatened by destructive feelings, its own and those it has projected onto its mother that it feels in danger of losing its good, loving mother entirely. The infant's solution to this danger has been to split the good mother off from the bad mother – as if, in the infant's imagination, they have become two separate mothers. In this way the good loving mother can remain idealised and perfect and not be contaminated by the wicked, hateful, bad mother.

We now move on to the second room in this imaginary art gallery. The pictures in this room represent the second stage of the infant's development. The infant is a few months older now. The first sequence of pictures shows us the inside of mother's body where the good, loving bits of her, and the bad, hating and hated bits of her, are jostling together. The infant's image of mother is changing, she is becoming a whole, separate and recognisable person. Nevertheless, the infant looks worried; recognising mother as a separate person has aroused new anxieties. If mother, whom the infant is entirely dependent on, is a separate person, the infant cannot control her, which means it is possible to lose her. This anxiety about dependency and fear of losing her generates renewed feelings of guilt, distress and the desire to put right the loved mother who, in the infant's fantasy, it may have harmed, or may yet harm, with its destructive rages. Klein saw this stage as crucial to the development of our feelings of concern and responsibility for others. This stage is also the beginning of some of the most important requirements for love: our ability to empathise, our desire to make others happy and, crucially, our ability to cope with ambivalence – people are rarely all good or all bad, most of us are somewhere in between.

But don't get the impression that these turbulent and deeply disturbing emotions have been successfully resolved and the infant can now grow up to live happily ever after. If we look more carefully at these pictures in the second room, we will see that each of the earlier images, remain within them, like ghosts; all the accumulated fears and anxieties, the paranoia, the envy, the greed, the hatred and the rage, are still there lurking beneath the surface.

No one knows, not even Klein, what goes on in the mind of a baby. She based her theories partly on observation of baby's dramatically fluctuating emotional states, and on her analysis of the imaginative world of young children, paying attention to their dreams and nightmares and the highly dramatic stories they invent when playing. Children's play stories often involve major conflicts between characters or animals who are thinly disguised representations of important people in the child's life, parents, siblings or whoever. The child is like a little theatre director in charge of all the parts in the dramas, casting its self, its toys, other children or adults as the good or the wicked, the ones who punish, tear apart, get rid of and destroy and the ones who magically rescue and restore to life.

What is striking about Klein's analysis of the emotional world of babies and young children is how the psychodynamic processes she describes are recognisable in many adult love-hate relationships. In *Mothering Psychoanalysis* (1991), Janet Sayers describes how the anxieties about the dreaded prospect of losing mother, which arise because of recognising her as a separate person, typically manifests itself in two-year olds:

> the child regularly seeks to ward off these anxieties by manically cultivating an attitude of contempt and denigration towards the mother as someone whose loss would not cause it any pain. This involves denying its dependence on her – a denial that is particularly obvious in the vehement and omnipotent tantrum protests of two-year olds.

I think the similarity between this description of the behaviour of two-year-old infants and the behaviour of some adults in the grips of an abusive, hate-filled rage is striking. Klein noted that this struggle between love and hate continues throughout our emotional lives and profoundly influences our adult love relationships.

We are all on an emotional continuum from white to black, from love to hate, from idealisation to denigration – only for most of us most of the time our feelings of love and hate are fluctuating in the various shades of grey. We develop an ability to accept our ambivalent feelings; we recognise that our loved one is neither an idealised model of perfection nor a monster. We regulate our emotions and empathise with the person we love, even if at times the struggle between the love and the hate we feel is hard to bear, even if there are times when we long to punish them and hurt them, we restrain ourselves and maintain our respect for their autonomy. But for some people, particularly in adult love relationships when anxieties about dependency are reawakened, their picture of their loved one can oscillate more wildly between an idealised image of perfection and a despised object of hatred. For them their all-consuming destructive state of rage – like that of the monstrous, hate-filled, green-eyed baby – obliterates all other feelings or concerns including their ability to empathise with the hated love object. The result, as Melanie Klein observed, 'is liable to become a source of danger in human relationships.'

Kleinian portraits of two men in my life

My father never hit my mother. He never allowed himself to cross that line: he never lost his moral faculties, his sense of right and wrong. Nevertheless, my father's occasional rages with my mother were dark episodes fuelled by an intense and frightening hatred. Occasionally his hatred was ejected in a stream of cruel words like spitting arrows, but mostly his rage was withheld behind a cold, hard wall of silence.

On the other hand, when he wasn't hating my mother his world revolved around loving her; he put her on a pedestal and idealised her, he provided for her, looked after her, cosseted her and attended to all her demands. My mother gloried in his attentiveness. We children were never in doubt that my mother was the most loved and most important person in our house and her needs always came first, except when my father was in a walled-in silent rage.

It's not difficult to see the schizoid and paranoid tendencies in my father. He was splitting my mother – denigrating her when he was angry and hated her and idealising her and pampering her as a way of expressing his remorse and his eagerness to make amends. Pampering her was also a way of possessing and controlling her; he needed to make her dependent on him as a defence against his anxiety about his own dependency on her. But at times his need for her became suffocating and unbearable, so much so that he wanted to hurt her. He would then become afraid of the terrible things that in his rage he had imagined. His self-imposed exile, and his walled-in angry silence, were ways of protecting her and himself from the dangerous destruction his rage might unleash and the awful consequences that might ensue; that he might destroy her or worse, he might lose her. The thought of losing her made him feel as if his entire world was disintegrating. He then became flooded with feelings of guilt and remorse. It was imperative that he tell her he was sorry and make everything alright again, before it was too late, and he lost everything he loved.

The effect on me as a small child witnessing his walled-in rage and my mother's helpless tears was also complicated. My brother had learnt to skilfully absent himself from difficult emotional situations. But my mother expected my sister and I to take her side, to feel sorry for her, to look after her and be angry with our father on her behalf. My sister, probably because she was the eldest, dutifully took on the role. But I couldn't blame my father. Instead I thought he was lonely and unhappy in his walled-in rage, I felt sorry for him and wanted to save him, but I didn't know how.

It's no accident that my favourite fairy tale was *Beauty and the Beast*. Beauty was special because she was good, unlike her nasty stepmother and envious sisters who were selfish, narcissistic and unkind. Beauty even sacrificed herself to save her beloved father's life by going to Beast's castle in her father's place. She saw that beneath Beast's terrifying rampages he was lonely and distressed. She transferred her love for her father onto Beast and in response to her courage, love and devotion Beast magically transformed into the handsome prince of her dreams.

What pernicious propaganda on behalf of Beasts everywhere! Beauty was just a girl locked away in a cold, draughty castle with a rampaging Beast – of course she would not have been able to save him.

When I was in my twenties, I fell in love with Harry, a man with a razzle-dazzle kind of charm. We found a flat together and for a short while I believed I was happy. There were signs that something was seriously wrong very early in our relationship, but I refused to see what I didn't want to see. Couples fight and there are times when they hate each other – that's what I told myself. I didn't want my dream shattered.

Harry's rages would usually begin with a trivial domestic crime I had supposedly committed. At first, they were furious verbal attacks. I would shout back, and sometimes these furious spats would end in both of us laughing. But on other occasions this would further inflame him, and his rages became violent, usually ending with him flinging my clothes into a bag demanding that I leave. He would then become filled with remorse; he was sorry, he didn't know what had come over him, he couldn't live without me, he promised to change. I believed him. I even pretended to myself that I could save him. I thought I could cure the beast in him through love.

Harry had learnt his bullying behaviour from his father, a controlling bully who had expected excellence and perfection from his only son. Harry's mother once told me that all the men in his father's family had had a terrible temper. Yet sometimes, when I watched him raging, I felt strangely detached. I had a strong feeling that it wasn't me or his father he was raging at; it was his mother he was seeing in his mind's eye.

Why didn't I confide in my family or friends? I think it was because I was ashamed; I didn't want to be a victim. It took me a long time to admit the truth even to myself. Decades after our relationship ended, I trained as a psychotherapist. It was then that I recognised aspects of Harry's behaviour in Melanie Klein's description of the infant's paranoid-schizoid rage with its mother. Like the Kleinian infant, after his destructive rampage had burnt out, Harry would flip into a state of remorse, regret and a child-like terror that I was going to leave him. Having been the most hated person who had to be destroyed, I was now the most loved, needed, idealised person he could not live without. Normal life would resume, the rages were forgotten, until the next episode.

Looking back, I can see how dangerous my Oedipal fixation was. Like Beauty in the fairy tale, I had transferred my childhood need to save my father onto my partner. What's more, Harry also offered me something that my father could never give me. I never knew what was really going on within my father's hidden emotional world. In contrast, Harry shot out all his feelings as if from an emotional blunderbuss. At least I knew what was going on in his messed up interior world – or I thought I did. Also, in a way Harry gave me the opportunity to express my own rage: I could have the fight I was never able to have with my father, as if by proxy. But finally, ours was never the fight between equals I pretended it was. Harry wasn't a two-year-old child; he was a man and he crossed the line.

I was lucky. Whilst my Oedipal fixation may have lured me into the relationship with Harry, my father's love and respect also gave me the ego strength I needed to survive this toxic relationship.

I had learnt from my father's self-restraint that there are moral boundaries in relationships that neither men nor women should ever cross.

Why some women return to their abuser

The Spanish film *Take My Eyes* (2003) is a vivid portrayal of domestic violence. In the film Pilar, a young wife, after suffering years of violence at the hands of her husband, Antonio, flees her home with her young son. She stays with her sister and begins to make a new life for herself. But Antonio is determined to win her back; he attends a programme of cognitive behavioural therapy and anger management for men who abuse their partners. When he has nearly completed the course, he finds Pilar and assures her that this time, with the help of therapy, he really has changed. He promises he will never hurt her again and begs her to fetch their little boy and they can go home together as a family. This is what Pilar has been longing for. She relents, and they go home.

The next morning Pilar puts on a pretty dress to wear for a job interview she has at the local art gallery. Antonio is in the sitting room looking though the catalogue of the gallery's classical art collection which Pilar has left on the table. A painting of a nude woman catches his eye, he becomes increasingly agitated. Soon he has worked himself up into a full-scale fit of rage. He grabs Pilar as she is preparing to leave for the interview and tears off her dress. Not content with that, he strips her naked except for her bra and throws her out onto the balcony of their apartment. Pilar cowers pitifully, trying to cover her naked genitals with her hands; she's terrified that someone in the street below will look up and see her. She begs him to let her back in. Finally, he slides open the glass door, drags her back into the room and places his hands around her throat as if he is going to strangle her. Pilar is so terrified she wets herself. Antonio backs off and watches her with a cold mixture of fascination and disgust. He turns and walks out of the apartment.

What this scene shows with uncompromising honesty is how, when Antonio is in the grips of his rage, he is entirely devoid of any empathy for the woman he loves. His hatred consumes him. He imagines she is to blame for his violence because of what he believes she has done to him. She deserves to be punished for not loving him properly, for making him feel bad about himself, for humiliating him, for being the cause of all his unbearable feelings. He is determined to make her feel all the terrible things that he believes, in his mad rage, she has made him feel. This is his way of getting rid of all those bad feelings and feeling good about himself again. And the more he bullies and humiliates her the more self-righteous, grandiose and powerful he feels; it's like a drug, he's high on his own power over her body and her sexuality.

Some men, particularly those with narcissistic personality disorder, may attend the cognitive behavioural therapy and anger management courses as manipulative ploy to get their partner back. But the film's portrayal of Antonio tells us that he really did want to change. In fact, when he convinces Pilar he has changed, he almost certainly believes it too. But tragically, when he is in a jealous rage he is totally out of control. The cognitive behavioural therapy and anger management courses have not touched his personality disorder, which is notoriously difficult to treat.

People who try to help victims of domestic violence, such as therapists, social workers and even the police, sometimes complain that they cannot understand why some women repeatedly return to their abuser. Most women who go back, return because they are desperate. They have no money, they have children to look after and they have nowhere else to go. Also, many women are like Pilar: they still love their partners, and they long to be back in their own home with their own family. But for some women the dynamic of their relationship with their abuser is comparable to a dangerous addiction; it is as difficult to break free, and its hold over them can be just as deadly.

The abuse cycle goes something like this: two people fall in love. They project onto each other their fantasy ideal partner. Together they wrap themselves in a cocoon of glorious sex and mutual admiration. All the bad is projected onto the outside world. In their cocoon, life is perfect.

After a while the cocoon becomes airless and stifling. Typically, he becomes suspicious of her: he can't trust her, she doesn't love him properly, he only sees her faults, or he's insanely jealous, convinced she's really thinking about another man. His manner becomes increasingly paranoid, manic, grandiose and omnipotent. His hatred and his rage builds and builds. This rage is reminiscent of the inconsolable infant described by Melanie Klein. He has split the woman he loves into two. Whereas she was the idealised 'good mother', now all he can see is the hated 'bad mother' who won't, or can't, give him everything he wants. He attacks her, he wants to destroy her.

She is undoubtedly his victim, but at the same time she is also high on his enormous rage. When a woman is being violently abused, she naturally experiences her own intense feelings of rage and hatred and has her own fantasies of hurting or even killing her abuser, although the woman is usually physically weaker than the man and too terrified to act out her fantasies. But his fury allows her own infantile rage expression. For some women, the release of their own rage can be exciting. It taps into their childhood rage with their parent who neglected, abused or failed to protect them.

The final part of the abuse cycle is characterised by remorse and reparation. Typically, his rage burns out, he becomes very afraid of what he has done to her, and terrified of losing her. He sees her once more as the 'good mother'. He's like a helpless, crying infant desperate for her forgiveness, desperate to reassure her that he will never hurt her again, desperate for her to come home. She is hugely relieved. In a way, this is the moment she has wanted all her life. At last she has the love she once longed for from her father or mother. At last she has the reassurance that she is the only person in the world whom he loves and desires, and she is the only one who knows how to love him and understand him and save him from himself.

However toxic, these intense emotions fuelled by the adrenalin rush of excitement and terror, function like a powerful drug. This is why these extremes – from idealised love to murderous hate and back to idealised love again – can be so dangerously addictive.

One woman told me that she had been meeting her ex-boyfriend secretly at night. Their clandestine meetings had to be in secret because, after a particularly violent attack when she had called the police, the court had issued a restraining order to prevent him from attempting to see her again. She said she knew it was crazy, but she had been missing him terribly. She hated being on her own. She also missed the sex, she added in a whisper. I asked, what it was about the sex she missed? She was deeply ashamed to tell me this, but she had wondered if she was masochistic, for her pain made the sex more intense. It gave her a feeling of ecstasy as if she were completely losing herself in the sex and that was an incredible relief from the unbearable feeling of longing to be loved. This woman's childhood had been blighted by her father's violent rages when he would trash the house and threaten to cut her mother up into little pieces. She also recalled her father coming to her in tears, begging her forgiveness. He was sorry he had frightened her.

Another woman who repeatedly returned to her violent partner explained it this way. She and her partner were alike. They had both grown up in violent, alcohol-sodden households. Neither of them had parents who had loved and protected them, so they tried to look after each other. But they were both so damaged they ended up hurting each other. They were also the only ones who really understood each other in a world full of 'normal, undamaged people'. She looked at me accusingly. I knew she saw me as one of the 'normal people' who couldn't possibly understand her and why she was in love with a man who had attacked her so violently. When she first came to see me, I was the therapist whom she hoped would help her stay away from him, but a few months later I had become the enemy who was trying to prevent her going back to him.

One day she received a text from him telling her not to get in touch because he was in a new relationship. In therapy she became silent. She said she was depressed, suicidal. She said she didn't believe he was in love with someone else. She was still afraid that he would come back and kill her. But I thought she was more afraid that he wouldn't come back, that this really was the end of their relationship. This was hard for her to hear. She admitted, through her tears, that now she felt completely abandoned, as if she was falling apart, life without him, everything, was now pointless, completely meaningless.

Another woman furiously attacked me when I attempted to support the strong woman part of her that I thought could resist returning to the boyfriend who had abused her. She said she hated being called 'strong' and she 'hated ball-breaking feminists', she thought they were unattractive and horrible. She liked being feminine because 'men prefer feminine women.' I felt bewildered; where had this attack come from? It was only later when I realised that my attempt to get her to think again about returning to her abusive partner had brought her face-to-face with the unbearable feeling of fragmentation, emptiness and the abandonment she most feared. She was also angry with me because therapy had led her into a contradiction. She hated feeling powerless, but, at the same time, she desperately wanted to return to the familiar, self-destructive, victim position. I thought she was also, unconsciously, very afraid of her own powerful destructive impulses. Her fury with me was fuelled by her fury with her mother who had failed to protect her from her abusive father. But if she lifted the lid on her inner Pandora's box filled with hate, rage and envy, who knows what would happen!

David Celani, an American clinical psychologist, worked extensively with women victims of domestic violence. In *The Illusion of Love: Why the Battered Woman Returns to Her Abuser* (1994), Celani provides a brilliant analysis of the psychology of domestic abuse. He builds on the psychological model the Scottish psychoanalyst W.R.D. Fairbairn devised, based on his work with neglected and abused children in a care home (see page 78, Chaper 4). Celani realised that his clients who were addicted to the abuse cycle frequently had a history that was like that of the children Fairbairn had worked with. What's more, many of their abusers had also suffered from violence, abuse or neglect in their childhoods:

> When two character disordered people find each other, all the danger of experiencing their inner emptiness is banished by the alternation of intense hopefulness and abject despair. This is

> the basis of so many pathological partnerships. The character disordered individual may not be able to verbalise it, but she senses her similarly disordered partner understands her.

In short, what Celani is describing here is a fatal attraction.

Celani concluded that women return to their abuser for the same reason that Fairbairn's abused children desperately wanted to go home to their neglectful, abusive parents:

> they prefer abuse to the high anxiety of feeling abandoned and cut off from their identity. This is like the woman who is victim of her partner's abuse who prefers to return to her abuser than remain alone. She needs him to keep her identity intact.

In other words, the chaos, high drama, and adrenalin rush of extreme emotions have long been familiar to them. They have grown to need it to keep their identity intact. This is the hope they need to ward off despair. For them, this is what love is. These extremes of passionate love and violent hate are less frightening than the awful silence of being left alone, empty and abandoned.

A power struggle and the roots of misogyny

For millennia there has been a powerful undercurrent of misogyny in most societies. But what drives the unconscious dynamic of misogyny and its iron grip over culture and society? And why, despite recent advances in feminism, does misogyny remain so devilishly hard to shift?

The feminist Dorothy Dinnerstein thought Melanie Klein had discovered the roots of misogyny. In *The Mermaid and the Minotaur* (1976), she argued that if our unconscious image of woman is rooted in our infantile experience of mother in the paranoid-schizoid stage of infant development no wonder woman is feared; her nebulous, engulfing power is terrifying and overwhelming. This woman, whom we desire for nurture, comfort and love could just as easily smother us, tear us to pieces or swallow us up.

Dinnerstein constructs a compelling case for how this image of the all-powerful mother is to be found in the cultural unconscious of most societies. For example, her terrifying power resembles that of the goddesses of creation and destruction revered in the ancient cultures of Egypt and Greece and still worshipped in the form of the goddess Kali in the Hindu religion. It is interesting how to combat, contain and control the awesome power of this creator-destroyer woman, the monotheistic religions with their one male God employed the same psychological defence as that used by the infant: splitting.

Splitting is one of the most effective, age-old means of taking away women's power. The 'good women' – the mothers, wives, and good girls next door – are idealised and split off in a separate compartment, to prevent them being contaminated by the 'bad women' – sex objects, sluts, and whores – women who are bought and sold and used and abused according to man's bidding. These women are reviled, denigrated and secretly, or not so secretly, sexually desired. The most ubiquitous example of this is the splitting of woman into the virgin and the whore. Icons of the idealised Virgin Mary, as the perfect, de-sexed, benevolent mother with her contented baby on her lap are to be found throughout Christendom. She has been split off from Eve who was made responsible for man's fall from grace because of the dangerous temptation posed by her sexuality.

Klein agreed with Freud, that the Oedipus complex is an important stage in the sexual development of children. But if we take on board Klein's vision of the infant's deeply ambivalent feelings towards its mother in the earlier paranoid-schizoid stage of development, the implications of the Oedipal transition for boys are different than for girls. For both genders, the rage with their mother's power to give or withhold whatever they want whenever they want it, coexists with their love and dependency on her. But as we saw in Chapter 3, as the boy becomes aware of his gender, he realises he has a secret weapon, something his mother does not have: his much-prized penis. He is a male like his father, who also has a penis, and his father appears to have an exciting and different power than his mother's, if not in the family, then in the world of men beyond the family.

In other words, boys learn early that their masculinity is a defence against their fear of female power. As we have seen, men who abuse women typically have an intense and paranoid fear of feeling emasculated, impotent, powerless and dependent in their intimate relationships, as well as in the wider world. Their defence against their vulnerability is to use violence and intimidation in the home to regain their illusion that they are powerful and in control, and to bolster their grandiose demonstration of potency. I think this takes us to the heart of some men's misogyny. The man's dependency on the woman he loves and sexually desires arouses not only his fear that she might abandon him, but also a primitive rage against her power over him. If we add to this performance anxiety, worries about penis size, premature ejaculation and the vulnerability of the male genitals (which we saw in Chapter 2), his solution, to prove that he doesn't need her by attacking her and tossing her away, makes a kind of primitive sense. He's like an infant in a tantrum who throws his favourite toy out of the cot, and thereby, in his fantasy at least, he restores his own masculine power. Of course, after the infant has tossed away its favourite toy, it cries because it wants its mother to bring it back.

The male-dominated power hierarchy in so many societies and cultures has historically played a huge part in the different learned behaviours of men and women. Men who have grown up in a family where their father demonstrated his power through dominance and control, and in a culture where this kind of masculinity has been traditionally prized, are more likely to take for granted that sex is about fulfilling their own sexual needs, the women's pleasure comes second, if at all. Women who have grown up in similar circumstances are more likely to have learned, from their mothers and other women in their community, that her value lies in her sexuality and her ability to fulfil the man's desires; attending to her own sexual needs comes second, if at all. Not that all women are victims. Women's rage, hatred and envious attacks on men, women and their own children can be devastating.

Freud had something of a blind spot when it came to women's power. If the woman has any power, it is within the confines of her position as the object of desire. But not recognising that woman's power exists beyond the limitations of her sexual power is also the most effective way to render her powerless. Sadly, as we saw in Chapter 2, too many women believe that their power and even their identity depends on their appearance and how attractive they are to men. Many women also have an almost touching concern with looking after the man's vulnerable ego. Too often the price they pay is neglecting their own sexual needs and desires.

Dinnerstein, like Shere Hite, believed that the only effective means to moderate our unconscious ambivalence towards the mother, and by extension to women generally, lies in education and political change. She questioned gender stereotypes and argued passionately for childcare to be equally shared between the mother and the father, which she believed would diminish these distorted images of male and female power and eventually create a more equal society. She would be horrified to discover that children's toy shops are still filled with action men and guns for little boys and pink princess dresses and Barbie dolls for little girls.

I'm heartened by the fact that the millennial generation have revived the conversation about gender and sexuality. They are questioning outdated gender stereotypes and embracing role models that truly reflect the complex and rich diversity of gender and sexual identities. Feminism, embraced by men as well as women, has always provided the best hope for fulfilment in sexual relationships. However, the lesson of the last hundred years has been that the more power women achieve in both the political and personal spheres, the more some men fear losing their power, status and potency – hence the periodic backlashes against feminism. Deep change, whether it is psychological, social or political, is a long, slow and difficult process. But change is urgently needed.

> The early mother's apparent omnipotence, then, her ambivalent role as ultimate source of good and evil, is a central source of human malaise: our species' uneasy, unstable stance toward nature, and its uneasy, unstable sexual arrangements, are inseparable aspects of this malaise.
>
> (Dinnerstein 1976)

Afterword

The history of psychoanalysis has largely downplayed the importance of sex or ignored sex altogether. This seems odd, as Freud, the founding father of psychoanalysis, is most well known for being obsessed with sex. However, many psychotherapists and counsellors I have met over the years have told me they learnt very little about sex in their training institutes. The discoveries of the sexologists (Kinsey, Masters and Johnson, and Hite) certainly weren't included in their curriculums. If you were interested in sex, it was assumed that you would seek further training in psychosexual therapy with a view to specialist work with clients who seek help with the more complex and extreme sexual problems. The result, for therapists working with the kind of everyday problems that come up in their consulting rooms, is the assumption that asking about their client's sex life, if their client hasn't specifically mentioned sex, is intrusive. 'We don't want to be intrusive' has echoes of the classic excuse many parents use to avoid talking to their children about sex.

To put it another way, talking about sex can be difficult for therapists as well as our clients. In my experience, unless clients come to see you with a specific sexual problem, many clients find it too embarrassing to bring up sex. Or they assume their depression or anxiety, or even the problems they want to talk about in their relationship have little or nothing to do with sex. They may be right – their problems don't have anything to do with sex. It may also be that the subject of sex is just too difficult for them to bring up. It's too hard to face the powerful feelings of shame, embarrassment and inadequacy even in a psychotherapy session. This is why it is important for therapists to stop being coy about sex. If your client doesn't bring up sex, ask them gently, but ask them! If your training institute doesn't include training about sex, ask them to include it in the curriculum.

Recently I attended a psychosexual course where for half a day the participants, all qualified psychotherapists and counsellors, talked about their personal sexual histories. The participants were from a variety of different cultures, but the thing most of us had in common was that we had learnt very little about sex in our childhood families. Most of what we had learnt, not to mention the words we had picked up about sex from other children, was relentlessly negative or just plain wrong. Our discussion moved on to how these negative attitudes towards sex had impacted on our own sexual histories. Spending a morning talking about sex, and sharing our stories, was at times sad and disturbing, but it was also incredibly interesting, and the session was full of vitality.

The big lesson for all of us, professional therapists and counsellors as well as our clients, is that talking about sex need not be embarrassing or shameful, rather it is hugely rewarding and central to our own well-being as well as to the well-being of our clients.

Acknowledgements

This book could never have been written without all my clients who have taught me so much over the years. But most of all, I owe a huge debt of gratitude to my ex-clients who have given me their permission to share their stories of the work we did together for this book. I want to thank Danielle Kerris for reading each draft of the manuscript and bolstering me with her enthusiasm as well as her valuable feedback. Thanks also to my UK colleagues Brian Solts, Anne Marie Salm, and Carmen O'Leary, and to Bracha Hadar in Israel and Saeunn Kjartansdottir in Iceland, who have all given me their warm support. I want to give a big thank you to Sylvia Hutchinson for her patient, wise and caring supervision. Thanks also for the huge amount I learnt from my training group therapist, Jane Campbell, Inge Hudson and all my teachers and colleagues at the Turvey Institute for Group-Analytic Psychotherapy. Many thanks also for the many learning opportunities provided by the Institute of Group Analysis, the Tavistock Clinic and Tavistock Relationships. Thanks also to Kerry Boettcher at Wordnoodle. And many thanks to my editor Russell George for his enthusiasm and encouraging feedback as I completed the manuscript for publication.

Finally, I would like to thank my husband Brian for reading my many revisions with a fine-tooth comb, and my stepson Stephen who encouraged me from the outset to write this book because he 'wanted to read it.' Tragically, Stephen died before the manuscript was completed, but his unerring belief in the value of this project and his unstinting love and support stay with me.

References

Ainsworth, M., Blehar, M., Eaters, E., Wall, S. (1979) *Patterns of Attachment: A Psychological Study of the Strange Situation* London: The Psychology Press.

Annie Hall (1977) Screenplay and director Woody Allen. New York, United Artists Corporation.

Austen, J. (1813) *Pride and Prejudice* Letchworth: The Temple Press Letchworth.

Bodenheimer, D. (2010) Sandor Ferenczi: A Life Lived Dyadically, *Psychoanalytic Social Work*, Vol. 17, No. 1, pp. 17–29.

Bonomi, A. (2013) 'Double Crap!' Abuse and Harmed Identity in Fifty Shades of Grey, *Journal of Women's Health*, Vol. 22, No. 9.

Bowlby, J. (1973) *Separation: Anxiety and Anger* London: Pimlico.

Bowlby, J. (1988) *A Secure Base* Hove: Brunner-Routledge pp. 50, 55.

Celani, D. (1994) *The Illusion of Love: Why the Battered Woman Returns to Her Abuser* New York: Columbia University Press pp. 142–145.

Dinnerstein, D. (1976) *The Mermaid and the Minotaur: Sexual Arrangements and the Human Malaise* New York: Other Press p. 100.

Fairbairn, W.R.D. (1952) *Psychoanalytic Studies of the Personality* London: Routledge and Keegan Paul.

Fonagy, P. (2001) *Attachment Theory and Psychoanalysis* London: Karnac p. 10.

Fraley, C., Shaver, P. (2000) Adult Romantic Attachment: Theoretical Developments, Emerging Controversies and Unanswered Questions, *Review of General Psychology*, Vol. 4, No. 2, pp. 132–154.

Freud, S. (1899) *Interpretation of Dreams* London: Penguin p. 364.

Freud, S. (1905a) *Infantile Sexuality* (*Three Essays on the Theory of Sexuality and Other Works*) London: Penguin p. 123.

Freud, S. (1905b) *The Sexual Aberrations* (*Three Essays on the Theory of Sexuality and Other Works*) London: Penguin pp. 71–75.

Freud, S. (1905c) *Transformations of Puberty* (*Three Essays on the Theory of Sexuality and Other Works*) London: Penguin p. 149.

Freud, S. (1909) *Analysis of a Phobia in a Five-Year-Old Boy (The 'Wolfman' and Other Cases)* London: Penguin 2002.

Freud, S. (1912) *On the Universal Tendency to Debasement in the Sphere of Love (Three Essays on the Theory of Sexuality and Other Works)* London: Penguin pp. 247, 255, 259.

Freud, S. (1918) *The Taboo of Virginity (Three Essays on the Theory of Sexuality and Other Works)* London: Penguin p. 277.

Freud, S. (1925) *Some Psychical Consequences of the Anatomical Distinction Between the Sexes (Three Essays on the Theory of Sexuality and Other Works)* London: Penguin p. 337.

Freud, S. (1930) *Civilisation and Discontents* London: Penguin p. 25.

Gathorne-Hardy, J. (2005) *Kinsey, a Biography* London: Pimlico p. 253.

Hall, P. (2013) *Understanding and Treating Sex Addiction* Hove: Routledge pp. 33–49.

Hite, S. (1976) *The Hite Report, a Nationwide Study of Female Sexuality* edition published 1977 in the British Commonwealth by Summit Books pp. 60, 130–131, 157, 194–196, 199–200, 226, 232, 258–259, 262, 332–337.

Hite, S. (1981) *The Hite Report on Male Sexuality* London: Macdonald Optima pp. 338–343, 355–357, 369–376.

Hite, S. (2005) *Oedipus Revisited* London: Arcadia Books p. 37.

James, E.L *Fifty Shades of Grey* (2011) Vintage Books London.

Jamieson, L. (2004) *The State of Affairs: Explorations in Infidelity and Commitment* edited by Duncombe, J., Harrison, K., Allan, G., Marsden, D. Mahwah, NJ: Lawrence Erlbaum Associates pp. 36–37.

Jelinek, E. (Novel 1993) *The Piano Teacher* London: Serpent's Tail Classics.

Jung, C. (1907) *The Freud/Jung Letters* Princeton, NJ: Princeton University Press 1974 p. 95.

Kinsey, A., Gebhard, P., Pomeroy, W. (1954) *Sexual Behaviour in the Human Female* Bloomington, IN: Indiana University Press.

Kinsey, A., Pomeroy, B., Martin, C. (1948) *Sexual Behaviour in the Human Male* Vol One New York: Ishi Press International pp. 180–181, 164.

Klein, M. (1928) *Early Stages of the Oedipus Complex (Love, Guilt, Reparation and Other Works 1921–1945)* London: Vintage p. 197.

Klein, M. (1937) *Love, Guilt and Reparation* (from *Love, Guilt and Reparation and Other Works*) London: Vintage 1998 pp. 308–313.

Lawrence, D.H. (1928) *Lady Chatterley's Lover* London: Penguin Classics.

Lee, H. (1996) *Virginia Woolf* (from *'Sketch of the Past'* in *Moments of Being* edited by Schulkind, J. revised 1985) London: Chatto and Windus pp. 80, 125–126.

Le Faye, D. (1996) *Jane Austen's Letters* Oxford: Oxford University Press p. 221.

Lloyd, E. (2005) *The Case of the Female Orgasm* Cambridge, MA: Harvard University Press.

Lundberg, F., Farnham, M. (1947) *Modern Woman: The Lost Sex* New York: Harper and Brothers Publishers.

Masters, W.H., Johnson, V.E. (1970) *Human Sexual Inadequacy* New York: Bantam Books p. 218.

Moore, A. (2009) Relocating Marie Bonaparte's Clitoris, *Journal: Australian Feminist Studies*, Vol. 24, No. 60: Genital Modification, pp. 149–165.

The Piano Teacher film (2001) Screenwriter and director Michael Haneke Curzon Artificial Eye.

Potter, C. (2004) Why Do We Still Fall for Mr Darcy?, *The Guardian Newspaper*.

Rudnytsky, P. (2002) *Reading Psychoanalysis* Ithaca, NY: Cornell University Press p. 132.

Sayers, J. (1986) *Sexual Contradictions: Psychology, Psychoanalysis, and Feminism* London: Tavistock Publications p. 56.

Sayers, J. (1991) *Mothering Psychoanalysis* London: Penguin.

Secunda, V. (1993) *Women and Their Fathers* London: Cedar p. 256.

Take My Eyes (2003) Screenplay Icíar Bollaín and Alicia Luna, director Icíar Bollaín Spain: Alta Films.

Wismeijer, A.J., van Assen, M.A.L.M. (2013) Psychological Characteristics of BDSM Practitioners, *The Journal of Sexual Medicine*, Vol. 10, No. 8.

Woolf, V. (1927) *To the Lighthouse* London: Grafton Books.

Woolf, V. (1931) *Professions for Women* (*Women and Writing*) London: The Women's Press p. 59.

Young, L., Alexander, B. (2012) *The Chemistry between Us: Love, Sex and the Science of Attraction* London: Penguin Random House.

Index